Lust

Pride
Michael Eric Dyson

Envy
Joseph Epstein

Anger
Robert A. F. Thurman

Sloth
Wendy Wasserstein

Greed
Phyllis A. Tickle

Gluttony
Francine Prose

Lust
Simon Blackburn

For over a decade, the New York Public Library and Oxford University Press have annually invited a prominent figure in the arts and letters to give a series of lectures on a topic of his or her choice. Subsequently these lectures become the basis of a book jointly published by the Library and the Press. For 2002 and 2003 the two institutions asked seven noted writers, scholars, and critics to offer a "meditation on temptation" on one of the seven deadly sins. *Lust* by Simon Blackburn is the third book from this lecture series.

Previous books from the New York Public Library/Oxford University Press Lectures are:

The Old World's New World by C. Vann Woodward
Culture of Complaint: The Fraying of America by Robert Hughes
Witches and Jesuits: Shakespeare's Macbeth by Garry Wills
Visions of the Future: The Distant Past, Yesterday, Today, Tomorrow
by Robert Heilbroner
Doing Documentary Work by Robert Coles
The Sun, the Genome, and the Internet by Freeman J. Dyson
The Look of Architecture by Witold Rybczynski
Visions of Utopia by Edward Rothstein, Herbert Muschamp,
and Martin E. Marty

Also by Simon Blackburn

Being Good: An Introduction to Ethics
Think: A Compelling Introduction to Philosophy
Ruling Passions: A Theory of Practical Reasoning
The Oxford Dictionary of Philosophy
Essays in Quasi-Realism
Spreading the Word: Groundings in the Philosophy or Language

Edited Works

Meaning, Reference, and Necessity (editor)
Truth (with Keith Simmons)

Lust

The Seven Deadly Sins

Simon Blackburn

The New York Public Library

UNIVERSITY PRESS

2004

OXFORD
UNIVERSITY PRESS

Oxford   New York
Auckland   Bangkok   Buenos Aires   Cape Town   Chennai
Dar es Salaam   Delhi   Hong Kong   Istanbul   Karachi   Kolkata
Kuala Lumpur   Madrid   Melbourne   Mexico City   Mumbai   Nairobi
São Paulo   Shanghai   Taipei   Tokyo   Toronto

Published by Oxford University Press, Inc.
198 Madison Avenue, New York, New York 10016

www.oup.com

Oxford is a registered trademark of Oxford University Press

Library of Congress Cataloging-in-Publication Data
Blackburn, Simon.
Lust : the seven deadly sins / Simon Blackburn
p. cm.
Based on a lecture series in the humanities hosted by the
New York Public Library.
Includes bibliographical references.
ISBN 0-19-516200-5
1. Lust—religious aspects—Christianity.
I. Title.
BV4627.L8B5852004
176—dc21

Book design by planettheo.com

9 8 7 6 5 4 3 2 1
Printed in the United States of America
on acid-free paper

Contents

Editor's Note

This volume is part of a lecture and book series on the Seven Deadly Sins cosponsored by the New York Public Library and Oxford University Press. Our purpose was to invite scholars and writers to chart the ways we have approached and understood evil, one deadly sin at a time. Through both historical and contemporary explorations, each writer finds the conceptual and practical challenges that a deadly sin poses to spirituality, ethics, and everyday life.

The notion of the Seven Deadly Sins did not originate in the Bible. Sources identify early lists of transgressions classified in the 4th century by Evagrius of Pontus and then by John of Cassius. In the 6th century, Gregory the Great formulated the traditional seven. The sins were ranked by increasing severity and judged to be the greatest offenses to the soul and the root of all other sins. As certain sins were subsumed into others and similar terms were used interchangeably according to theological review, the list evolved to include the seven as we know them: Pride, Greed, Lust, Envy, Gluttony, Anger, and Sloth. To counter these violations, Christian theologians classified the Seven Heavenly Virtues—the cardinal: Prudence, Temperance, Justice, Fortitude, and the theological: Faith, Hope, and Charity. The sins inspired medieval and Renaissance writers including Chaucer, Dante, and Spenser, who personified the seven in rich and memorable characters. Depictions grew to include associated colors, animals, and punishments in hell for the deadly offenses. Through history, the famous list has emerged in theological and philosophical tracts, psychology, politics, social criticism, popular culture, and art and literature. Whether the deadly seven to you represent the most common human foibles or more serious spiritual shortcomings, they stir the imagination and evoke the inevitable question— what is *your* deadly sin?

Our contemporary fascination with these age-old sins, our struggle against, or celebration of, them, reveals as much about our continued desire to define human nature as it does about our divine aspirations. I hope that this book and its companions invite the reader to indulge in a similar reflection on vice, virtue, the spiritual, and the human.

Elda Rotor

Preface

People presume each other to be acquainted with sin. So when the New York Public Library and Oxford University Press asked me to lecture on one of the Seven Deadly Sins, I was modest enough not to ask "Why me?" I did worry in case I got landed with sloth, not because of unfamiliarity with the vice, but because of doubts about having the energy to find something to say about it. Otherwise the field seemed wide open.

This essay grew—but not very much—out of my lecture. The sponsors might have asked a historian, or a theologian, but this is an essay by a philosopher. It is an essay about lust itself, but still more about ideas about lust. Those ideas have a history, some of which I try to exhibit, although this is not a work of history. The ideas also infuse our religious traditions, but although they were draped in religious clothing, we should not think of them as simply belonging to theology. As the historian Peter Brown, whose work I use in the book, nicely pointed out, in the 1960s the theology section of the great Oxford bookshop Blackwells lay through a corridor labeled "second-hand philosophy." It is people with ideas who try to work out what is the divine will, on this and every other matter, so by and large we can short-circuit the divine, and just look at the ideas.

It is usual to end a preface with a list of acknowledgments. Here I find myself baffled. A short list might arouse comment, and a long list would be worse still. Yet to thank nobody raises the suspicion that this is purely a work of armchair theory, a piece of furniture associated with only imperfect expressions of lust. Silence is my only option. But I would like to thank the two organizations I have already mentioned, and especially their representatives, Elda Rotor of Oxford University Press, and Betsy Bradley of the New York Public Library, for their support, first for the lecture, and then for this essay.

Lust

Introduction

We might fear that, as so often, Shakespeare got it right straight off:

> Th'expense of spirit in a waste of shame
> Is lust in action; and till action, lust
> Is perjured, murd'rous, bloody, full of blame,
> Savage, extreme, rude, cruel, not to trust,
> Enjoy'd no sooner but despised straight,
> Past reason hunted, and no sooner had
> Past reason hated, as a swallowed bait
> On purpose laid to make the taker mad;
> Mad in pursuit and in possession so,
> Had, having, and in quest to have, extreme;
> A bliss in proof, and proved, a very woe;
> Before, a joy proposed; behind, a dream.
>> All this the world well knows; yet none knows well
>> To shun the heaven that leads men to this hell.[1]

Broadminded though we take ourselves to be, lust gets a bad press. It is the fly in the ointment, the black sheep of the family, the ill-bred, trashy cousin of upstanding members like love and friendship. It lives on the wrong side of the tracks, lumbers around elbowing its way into too much of our lives, and blushes when it comes into company.

Some people like things a little on the trashy side.[2] But not most of us, most of the time. We smile at lovers holding hands in the park. But we wrinkle our noses if we find them acting out their lust under the bushes. Love receives the world's applause. Lust is furtive, ashamed, and embarrassed. Love pursues the good of the other, with self-control, concern, reason, and patience. Lust pursues its own gratification, headlong, impatient of any control, immune to reason. Love thrives on candlelight and conversation. Lust is equally happy in a doorway or a taxi, and its conversation is made of animal grunts and cries. Love is individual: there is only the unique Other, the one doted upon, the single star around whom the lover revolves. Lust takes what comes. Lovers gaze into each others' eyes. Lust looks sideways, inventing deceits and stratagems and seductions, sizing up opportunities (fig. 9). Love grows with knowledge and time, courtship, truth, and trust. Lust is a trail of clothing in the hallway, the collision of two football packs. Love lasts, lust cloys.

Lust subverts propriety. It stole Anna Karenina from her husband and son, and the besotted Vronsky from his honorable career. Living with lust is like living shackled to a lunatic. In Schopenhauer's splendid words, almost prophesying the Clinton presidency, lust is the ultimate goal of almost all human endeavour, exerts an adverse influence on the most important affairs, interrupts the most serious business at any hour, sometimes for a while confuses even the greatest minds, does not hesitate with its trumpery to disrupt the negotiations of statesmen and the research of scholars, has the knack of slipping its love-letters and ringlets even into ministerial portfolios and philosophical manuscripts.[3]

It might seem, then, quixotic or paradoxical, or even indecent, to try to speak up for lust. But that is what I shall try to do. The philosopher David Hume said that a virtue was any quality of mind "useful or agreeable to the person himself or to others."[4] Lust has a good claim to qualify. Indeed, that understates it, since lust is not merely useful but essential. We would none of us be here without it. So the task I set myself is to clean off some of the mud, to rescue it from the echoing denunciations of old men of the deserts, to deliver it from the pallid and envious confessors of Rome and the disgust of the Renaissance, to destroy the stocks and pillories of the Puritans, to separate it from other things that we know drag it down (for we shall find that there are worse things than lust, things that make pure lust itself impure), and so to lift it from the category of sin to that of virtue.

It is not a task to undertake lightly, and I have to ask questions of myself. Do I really want to draw aside the curtains and let light disperse the decent night that thankfully veils our embarrassments? Am I to stand alongside the philosopher Crates, the Cynic, who, believing that nothing is shameful, openly copulated in public with his wife Hipparchia?[5] Certainly not, but part of the task is to know why not.

Some might deny that there is any task left to accomplish. We are emancipated, they say. We live in a healthy, if sexualized, culture. We affirm life and all its processes. We have already shaken off prudery and embarrassment. Sex is no longer shameful. Our attitudes are fine. So why worry?

I find myself at one with many feminists in finding this cheery complacency odious, and not just because the expressions of a sexualized culture are all too often dehumanizing, to men and especially to women, and even to children.

The sexualization of our commercial culture is only a fascination with something that we fear or find problematic in many ways. When I lived in North Carolina, two- and three-year-old girls were usually made to wear bikini tops on the beach, and a six-year-old was banned from school because he attempted to kiss a fellow pupil. In some states, such as Georgia and Alabama, at least until recently, "any device designed or marketed as useful primarily for the stimulation of human genital organs" was regarded as obscene, and possession, sale, purchase, and so on were aggravated misdemeanors punishable by heavy fines and even prison time. (England is not much better: in England girls can legally have sex at 16 but cannot buy vibrators until they are 18.) When I gave the lecture, some 12 states had sodomy laws that applied to both heterosexual and homosexual couples—Alabama, Arizona, Florida, Idaho, Louisiana, Michigan, Massachusetts, Minnesota, North Carolina, South Carolina, Utah, and Virginia. Something similar was true of oral sex. While this book was in press the Supreme Court struck down Texas' anti-gay laws, keeping police at least a little farther out the bedroom (however with three justices dissenting). Like England, nearly all U.S. states deny prostitutes anything like adequate legal protection, in spite of the overwhelming social ills that the prohibition creates, in this field as in others.

Then on May 10, 2002, advised by John Klink, sometime strategist for the Holy See, the Bush administration refused to sign a United Nations declaration on children's rights unless the United Nation's current plans for sex and health education in the developing world were changed to teach that only sexual abstinence is permissible before marriage.

Within the United States, the federal government spends some $100,000,000 a year of American tax dollars on abstinence-only programs of sex education. This in spite of the fact that abstinence-only programs markedly increase young peoples' health risks by making sporadic, furtive, and unprotected copulations their only option. Human Rights Watch has issued a severe report on teenagers' rights to high-quality health and safety information, which is currently denied to them in schools.[6] A nice quote from a Texas teacher introduces the report: "Before [the abstinence-only program] I could say 'if you're not having sex, that's great. If you are, you need to be careful and use condoms.' Boy, that went out the window." The report notes that federal programs standardly lie to children, for example about the efficiency of condoms.

This is not, I think, the sign of a culture that has its attitudes to sexuality under control. Similarly in the United Kingdom, the Church of England is currently tearing itself apart over two issues. One is that of gay priests, and the other is that of women bishops. This, too, is not the sign of a culture in which sex is understood as it might be. So there is work to do.

But am I the right person to do it? When I gave the lecture in New York City from which this essay developed, I reflected upon no less than five disqualifications. First, there is my age. In terms of Titian's beautiful painting of the three ages of mankind, I inhabit the background, contemplating spiritual things (fig. 10). Nobody would be asked to give a lecture on lust until of an age when time and experience have blunted its fierce prick. Lust belongs with youth; middle age relies in greater part on memory or imagination. The young are naturally overcome by lust, but the middle-aged who show an undue interest in it are more likely to be accused of idle lechery. The sins of middle age are melancholy, envy, gluttony, and anger. By the time you are of an age to give a public lecture on lust, lust may have lost a little of its luster.

Second, I had to feel uncomfortable with my sex or gender. I am male, and for a long time now the discourse of sexuality, as the intelligentsia like to call it, has belonged to women and to other groups who feel they need to explain or justify themselves, notably gays. In the standard story, men are the oppressors, and grandfathers make strange bedfellows for victims and the marginalized. But part of my aim is to restore lust to humanity, and at least I can claim to be human.

Be that as it may, there is my third problem, which is my nationality. We English are renowned for our cold blood and temperate natures, and our stiff upper lips. When the poet Samuel Taylor Coleridge read the remark of a German writer, that dancing is an allegory of sexual love, he wrote indignantly that "In England, at least, our young Ladies think as little of the Dances representing the moods and manoeuvres of Sexual Passion as of the Man-in-the-Moon's whiskers; and woe be to the Girl who should so dance as to provoke such an interpretation." English passions include property and propriety, both enemies of lust. The nearest we are supposed to get to lust is something like Gainsborough's picture of Mr. and Mrs. Andrews, and one can easily imagine this prim couple saying what the paradigm Englishman Lord Chesterfield said of sex, that "the pleasure is momentary, the position ridiculous, and the expense damnable" (fig. 11).

Other nationalities are amazed that we English reproduce at all. One cannot imagine an Englishman lecturing on lust in France. We tend not to make a fuss. When witchcraft hysteria broke out in Europe in the sixteenth century and onward, a frequent accusation against women was that they had been copulating with the devil, who visited them in evil phallic form at night. But although we have the word for these nocturnal temptations, the incubus (and, even-handedly, one for the corresponding female visitor to men, the succubus), this charge was seldom made in English witchcraft trials. However, national pride requires me to note that, again unlike their continental counterparts, English witches seldom exerted their malevolent powers by making men impotent.[7]

The fourth problem I put to myself was what I anticipated, perhaps unfairly, about the audience. To the English, the American penchant for sharing a bed with each partner's lawyers, and after that with Jesus, feels uncomfortable. Five is a crowd, and we would be embarrassed, or even unmanned, by a ghostly audience distracting us with whispers of legal and religious proprieties. We like to lose ourselves, a notion which occupies us later.

Fifth, I had to lament my profession of philosopher, recalling the fate of my distinguished predecessor Bertrand Russell, who in 1941 was stripped of his appointment at the College of the City of New York, where he was to have taught logic. After a Catholic-inspired witch hunt he was dismissed on the grounds that his works were "lecherous, libidinous, lustful, venerous, erotomaniac, aphrodisiac, irreverent, narrow-minded, untruthful and bereft of moral fiber." For the record, occasionally he had suggested that the sexual mores of the 1930s were a little tyrannical, but his relevant writings were about logic, mathematics, and the theory of knowledge—the subjects he had been employed to teach.

In fact, there has always been something incongruous about the juxtaposition of philosophers and lust. There is a special pleasure to be had when we fall, as the medieval legend of Aristotle and Phyllis shows. The story was made up by one Henri d'Andeli, a thirteenth-century poet from Normandy. His poem, the *Lai d'Aristote*, tells how Alexander the Great, Aristotle's pupil, was lectured by the philosopher on the evils of spending too much time and energy on a courtesan, Phyllis. Alexander gave up Phyllis, but told her that this was upon Aristotle's advice. Phyllis vowed to get her revenge on Aristotle, which she did by singing and dancing and generally cavorting outside his study. "Her hair was loose, her feet were bare, and the belt was off her gown." Eventually Aristotle was snared, and, seizing Phyllis through the window, declared his passion to her. She consented to be his, provided he would first satisfy a little whim she had. He must let her saddle him and ride him around the garden. The besotted Aristotle did so, but not before Phyllis had summoned Alexander to witness the humiliation. "Master, can this be?" queried Alexander, whereupon Aristotle warned him that if lust can so overcome wisdom itself, a not-so-wise young man like Alexander must be doubly vigilant against it. In the story, Alexander sees the point and forgives Aristotle. There are many depictions of the scene in stained glass, tapestry, and paintings (fig. 1).

It is all completely apocryphal, telling us only about the medieval imagination and nothing about Aristotle. But it plugs into our sense that young, vigorous warriors and conquerors are suitable candidates for lust, not elderly philosophers. In the story, Phyllis takes Aristotle from contemplation to the worldly, a particularly poignant victory when book 10, the final book, of Aristotle's *Nicomachean Ethics* identifies contemplation as the highest activity of man. Also, Phyllis takes Aristotle out of his study to the garden, from the domain of reason to that of nature. There is an evident echo of the garden of Eden and the myth of the Fall. And Christian commentators of the time had no trouble giving the story a misogynistic turn, making Phyllis into Alexander's wife and supposing that the moral is not the victory of lust, but the deceitfulness of woman.

These five obstacles are indeed daunting. But the questions which lust, and still more our attitudes to lust, prompt are too interesting to leave aside. Apart from anything else, what a culture makes of "masculinity" or "femininity" spills into every corner of life. It determines how we grow up. It determines the script we follow, what people become proud about, and therefore by contrast what they are ashamed of or hostile toward. Our anxieties produce fantasies and distortion, aggression and ambition, violence and war. Fascism was perhaps the most obvious political movement that clustered around ideals of the Male, but it will not be the last. Islam's attitude to women and Western women need only be mentioned.

This is a small essay, but the landscape of human lust and human thinking about it is far too large to take in at a glance. People have devoted lifetimes to charting small parts of it. As I write, or you read, neurologists are plotting it, pharmacists are designing drugs to modify it, doctors are tinkering with its malfunctions, social psychologists are setting questionnaires about it, evolutionary psychologists are dreaming up theories of its origins, postmodernists are deconstructing it, and feminists are worrying about it. And a large part of the world's literature is devoted to it, or to its close relative, erotic love. I think of myself as no more than taking a philosophical stroll in the park, here and there stopping to point out an interesting view. The park is not a paradise. Weeds grow, serpents lie in wait, and people have built slums over parts of it. But we do not have to inhabit them, if we are careful.

CHAPTER ONE

Desire

It is not easy, to say the least, to identify the object of many of our desires. We are familiar with the idea that we may think we want one thing when we really want something else. We have grown used to the idea that we disguise our desires from ourselves, let alone from each other. Perhaps not our doings, nor our sayings, nor even the tales about ourselves we tell in our heads manifest our true desires. Ours is a suspicious age, receptive to the idea that our selves are slippery and mutable, many-layered, sometimes glimpsed but never known, more constructed than discovered. But this is not itself a new idea. Across the centuries a great deal of Christian energy went into spiritual disciplines designed to strip off the false veil of our deceptions and self-deceptions so as to reveal our true heart's desires underneath.

When we talk of lust it might seem clear enough what we are talking about: sexual desire. And it might seem equally obvious what that is. The boy and girl back from the bar, stumbling and stripping in the hall, tongues lolling and panting for "it," know what they want. It's simple enough. They want sex.

But that does not get to the heart of it. Someone might want sex for many reasons: to have children, to prove that they can do it, to gratify a partner, simply to be rid of someone, to advance their career, to provide a medical sample, or to earn some money. In such cases, they may desire sex without feeling lust; indeed in some of these cases absence of lust may be precisely the problem. Sex can be a means to further ends, and in any case biologically it is certainly there as a means to a further end, namely reproduction. Our boy and girl don't care about anything like that. Their frenzy is directed not at sexual activity as a means, but as an end in itself.

If we are biologically minded, we might say what they are really after is orgasm and the following relief. But that is clearly wrong. If he thinks about it at all, our boy may be dreading his orgasm as an unwanted terminus, an unwelcome interruption, a possible cause of humiliation and dissatisfaction. Or, he might fear that in spite of his partner's current enthusiasm, he is not going to get sex and may have to go and provide himself an orgasm later. And that is not what he wants. The focus of his lust is quite different. The mistake here is to confuse anything that brings desire to an end with the intended object of desire, the thing that is actually wanted. Bertrand Russell once proposed such a theory of desire, and it is implicit in the common psychological metaphor of "drives" aiming at their own "extinction." The philosopher Wittgenstein is supposed to have refuted Russell by pointing out that if Russell wanted food, his desire might be extinguished by a punch in the stomach. But Russell did not want a punch in the stomach. Our boy and girl do not want any old means to bring their desire to an end. Their parents' arrival might extinguish their desire very effectively, but it is not what they want.

Of course, orgasm itself might be wanted and often is. Indeed, it is fitting that it should be wanted. It is typically the ecstatic finale, and when we go to the theater we do not want to leave before the ecstatic finale. But neither is the ecstatic finale all we want, as if we could just make do with it, bypassing the rest of the performance. Nor do we only want the relief that follows the ecstatic finale, or the state of having been through it. We can have wants of that kind: I might not want to go to the dentist, but nevertheless want to enjoy the relief of having been to the dentist. I might be going to enjoy having been to the opera much more than I will enjoy enduring the opera. But that is because the processes are regarded as in themselves unpleasant, whereas our specimen boy and girl are anticipating nothing but pleasure.

A different attempt to delineate the matter biologically might identify lust simply with sexual arousal, a physical state that is relatively easy to identify, as well as making itself known to the subject. Unfortunately this is wrong, too. A person can certainly be in a state that would superficially be physically identifiable as arousal without feeling lust at all. Priapism is relatively rare, but is a naturally occurring state of men that leads to pain and embarrassment, not lust. And the same effect can be caused by injections of various chemicals into the penis. Excitements of various kinds can lead to physical arousal: some say traders on the stock exchange are particularly prone to it, but they need not be feeling sexual desire at the time. Physical arousal of this kind clearly has something to do with lust, but it is not enough. So we have to bring in the mind. Lust is a psychological state with a goal or aim. It wants to bring something about—but what?

Rather than saying that our boy and girl are just physically aroused, or that they want orgasm or relief, it is better to say that it is the whole play, the pleasure of sexual activity that is on their minds. But sexual activity encompasses many things—we can only guess at what might go on once they reach the bedroom—so we should talk not of pleasure, but of pleasures in the plural. Perhaps lust is essentially the anticipation of the pleasures of sexual activity.

Yet even that is not quite enough: imagine someone anticipating such pleasures, but somewhat ruefully. They might suffer from the melancholy feeling that their partner will manipulate them into feeling pleasure, when they would rather not, just as one might wish that one's boisterous friends would not drag one off to an evening in the bar, even if one anticipates enjoying it when one gets there. This is the reverse of lust. We have to specify that our couple desire what they anticipate.

By themselves, even desire for sexual activity and its pleasures, and desire for them as ends in themselves rather than strategic routes to something else, do not give us full-blown lust. Consider satiated libertines who regret the dying of the old fire. They desire to desire as they once did. In doing so, they also desire the activities and pleasures they once had: here, a desire to desire X implies a desire for X. They mourn the days, or nights, of arousal that are slipping into the past. But lust is not thereby electrified. It may remain mortifyingly absent. In the central cases we need to focus upon, lust is not only desire, but desire that is felt, the storm that floods the body, that heats and boils and excites. A cold desire does not count. We need to add the feelings, the portrait in the mind of the body's arousal.[8]

The earliest poems of desire in Western literature are those of Sappho, and she knew what she was talking about:

> whenever I catch
> sight of you, even if for a moment,

then my voice deserts me

and my tongue is struck silent, a delicate fire
suddenly races underneath my skin,

my eyes see nothing, my ears whistle like
the whirling of a top

and sweat pours down me and a trembling creeps over
my whole body, I am greener than grass
at such times, I seem to be no more than
a step away from death

but all can be endured, since even a pauper . . . [9]

We do not know what even a pauper can do, for tragically the fragment breaks off here.

The arousal, the flooding of the body, can be studied medically, by chemists, molecular biologists, and neurophysiologists. We are told for instance, that

The feelings of sexual desire are best understood as an emergent property of at least four interlocking physiological systems, at least eleven different regions of the brain, more than thirty distinct biochemical mechanisms, and literally hundreds of specific genes supporting these various processes. [10]

The interlocking systems are the nervous, endocrine, circulatory, and genitourinary systems. There are also autonomic sexual mechanisms that ignore the brain altogether. They underlie and contribute to the flooding of the body by desire. Their different functioning at different times and in different people will direct the intensity with which lust is felt, and their dormancy may give us good reason, against Freudians, for denying that sexual desire is in the air at all. If we integrate mind and brain as we should, then the Freudian vision of even the infant mind as a seething hotbed of unconscious lusts is revealed as the fantasy that it is. No excitement, no blood boiling, no lust. But our concern is lust in the human world, Sappho's lust, not the correlates of lust in the body and brain.

Putting it all together, we are talking about the enthusiastic desire, the desire that infuses the body, for sexual activity and its pleasures for their own sake, and from now on that is what we shall take lust to mean.

CHAPTER TWO

Excess

So far we have confined ourselves to sexual desire, but the word *lust* has wider application: lust for life, lust for gold, lust for power. Perhaps sexual desire should be carefully recognized as just one kind of desire among others. Saint Thomas Aquinas put to himself the objection that lust was not confined to sexual (venereal) matters:

It would seem that the matter of lust is not only venereal desires and pleasures. For Augustine says (*Confessions* ii, 6) that "lust affects to be called surfeit and abundance." But surfeit regards meat and drink, while abundance refers to riches. Therefore lust is not properly about venereal desires and pleasures.[11]

He also worried that lust had been defined by previous authority as "the desire of wanton pleasure." But then wanton pleasure regards not only venereal matters but also many others. Therefore lust is not only about venereal desires and pleasures.

Aquinas was right to worry about getting this part of the subject straight. In many lists of the Seven Deadly Sins, lust is replaced by *luxuria* or luxury. This is not an innocent mistake or confusion, but reflects the urge to inject something morally obnoxious into the definition. If we associate lust with excess and surfeit, then its case is already lost. But it is a cheap victory: excessive desire is bad just because it is excessive, not because it is desire. If we build the notion of excess into the definition, the desire is damned simply by its name. And the notion of excess is certainly in the wings (as sonnet 129 made plain). If we say that someone has a lust for gold, we imply more than that he simply wants money, like the rest of us. We imply that the want is disproportionate, or has expelled other interests. It is not just that gold puts a gleam into his eye, it is that nothing else does, or gold puts too bright a gleam. The gleam has turned into a monomania.

There are many dimensions of excess. A desire might be excessive in its intensity if, instead of merely wanting something, we are too much preoccupied by it or we are obsessed by it or pine for it or are unduly upset by not getting it. Differently, a desire might be excessive in its scope, as when someone wants not just power, but complete power, or not just gold, but all the gold there is. We have to admit that sexual desire could be excessive in either way. It might preoccupy someone too much, and it might ask for too much. Don Juan illustrates both the fault of excessive preoccupation and that of encompassing too many objects. Yet many men might be hard put to it to know whether they differ from him in both ways, or only in one. President Clinton is reported to have gone into therapy in order to "cure" his sexual "addiction," yet the problem on the face of it (if that is the right word) was not with the intensity of his desire, but with its wayward direction and his limp self-control. And why did these minor faults, a subject of mirth in the rest of the world, arouse such obsessive hostility in conservative America? After all, it has been known for a long time that more prostitutes fly into towns hosting Republican conventions than Democratic ones. Perhaps this sector of the American public does not like to think of its president, its God of War, stretched out in post-coital slump, victim of the calmly triumphant Venus, and with his weapons demoted to mere playthings (fig. 2).

If we talk of excess, it seems we ought to be able to contrast it with some idea of a just and proportionate sexuality: one that has an appropriate intensity, short of obsession but more than indifference, and directed at an appropriate object. People manage that, sometimes. Indeed, nature often manages it for us, in one respect, since eventually we calm down and go to sleep. So it would seem quite wrong to say that lust is in and of itself bound to be excessive. Indeed, when we are listless or depressed, or old and tired, we suffer from loss of appetite, too little lust, not too much. And after all, judged from our actual choices rather than our moralizing, we like lust well enough. Advertising agencies fall over themselves to suggest that their products enable us to excite lust in others, but nobody ever made a fortune from prescribing ways of making ourselves repulsive.

There is indeed another dimension in which lust might seem in and of itself excessive, admitting of no moderation. Eating relieves our desire for food, our hunger. And we dine together, eating and talking, or eating and reading the newspaper or watching the television. But the activity that relieves our lust typically blocks out other functions. It doesn't literally make us blind, even temporarily, and we would be quick to desist if the wrong visitor arrived, or if someone shouted "Fire!" But it is as close to ecstasy—to standing outside ourselves—as many of us get. As the body becomes flooded with desire, and still more as the climax approaches, it blots out much of the world. It fills our mental horizon. The brain requires a lot of blood, so there is a saying that men have two organs that require a lot of blood, but only enough for one at a time. There is a literal truth here, and not only about men, which is that sexual climax drives out thought. It even drives out prayer, which is part of the church's complaint about it.

Perhaps it does not have to be like that: there are records of Chinese voluptuaries who could dictate letters while coupled to their partners. It is certainly virtuoso, but deficient in at least one of the pleasures of exercising lust, which is the abandonment itself.

This abandonment deserves more than a moment's attention. It a good thing if the earth moves. There is no such thing as a decorous or controlled ecstasy, so we should not want to persecute lust simply because of its issue in extremes of abandon. Indeed, such experiences are usually thought to provide one of life's greatest goods, and a yardstick for others. Even in the rigid atmosphere of Catholic sanctity, the best that mystics could do by way of expressing their ecstatic communion with God or Christ was by modeling it upon sexual ecstasy. The metaphors are the same: in the ecstatic communion the subject surrenders, burns, loses herself, is made blind or even temporarily destroyed, suffering a "little death." When Saint Teresa of Avila talked of an "arrow driven into the very depths of the entrails and the heart," so that the soul does not "know either what is the matter with it or what it desires," and still more when she talks of the experience as a distress but one "so delectable that life holds no delight that can give greater satisfaction," it was not only Bernini who was driven to depict her in terms of orgasm (fig. 3). Her contemporaries, as well, were hard put to know whether this was the work of God or the devil, and it was a close call when they finally decided on the former.[12]

The interesting thing is the association of such a state with *communion* and with knowledge (compare the biblical equation between knowing someone and having sex with them). Hard-nosed philosophers are apt to look askance at incommunicable knowledge, and since the mystic's claim to know something that the rest of us do not seems unverifiable, it is easy to remain skeptical about it. However sensible that may be in the case of divine ecstasy, it is harder to dismiss the association in the case of sexual ecstasy. Are all sexual experiences of communion, of being one, of becoming a kind of fusion of persons, to be dismissed? Is it illusion all the way down?

We shelve this for the moment, returning to Aquinas's own answer to the problem of definition. It is scarcely reassuring:

> As Isidore says . . . "a lustful man is one who is debauched with pleasures." Now venereal pleasures above all debauch a man's mind. Therefore lust is especially concerned with such like pleasures.[13]

First of all, it seems wrong to say that a lustful man is one who is debauched with pleasure: he may or may not be, depending on his luck. And in any case, sexual desire is rather more acute just when we are not debauched with pleasure. A sated man or woman is no longer lustful. And then the word "debauch" is scarcely neutral, implying riot and ruin. Finally, it is not true either that venereal pleasures debauch a man's mind. Newton seems to have been fairly ascetic, but Einstein was certainly not.

So we must not allow the critics of lust to intrude the notion of excess, just like that. We no more criticize lust because it can get out of hand, than we criticize hunger because it can lead to gluttony, or thirst because it can lead to drunkenness.

CHAPTER THREE

Two Problems
from Plato

At the beginning of the Western world, and in spite of the shining example of Sappho, Greek philosophers expressed wariness of sex. Pythagoras said that the best time for a man to make love is when he wants to weaken himself. Hippocrates, the father of medicine, and later on Plato as well, thought that sexual activity, the squandering of seed, involved a dangerous loss of energy. The Hippocratic writings also suggest that adolescent wet dreams are the precursor of insanity, a view that persisted at least until the nineteenth century, when it reached hysterical proportions.[14] And a variety of ills were laid at lust's door:

> Those who are bald are so because their constitution is phlegmatic: for during intercourse the phlegm in their heads is agitated and heated, and impinging upon the epidermis burns the roots of their hair, so that the hair falls out.[15]

In the fifth century B.C., Hesiod said that Eros has a power that is the enemy of reason, and this is perhaps an example.

In case we think that these attitudes are inevitable, doing no more than reflect universal facts of the human condition, we might want to contrast Eastern traditions of the rejuvenating and life-giving powers of lust. In the Eastern Han dynasty (A.D. 25–220), Taoists proposed a theoretical basis for immortality through sex. Indeed, one of the Taoist manuals asserted that the Yellow Emperor became immortal after having had sexual relations with twelve hundred women, although it seems probable that the number twelve hundred is more accurate than the claim of immortality. The sage Peng Tsu, by means of making love to ten to twenty girls every single night, was able to live to a good old age. Unfortunately it is not recorded how long the girls lived.

This is not the way the West took. One of the most famous images in philosophy is Plato's model of the soul in terms of the charioteer with his two horses. In the dialogue *Phaedrus* they are vividly described:

The one in the better position has an upright appearance, and is clean-limbed, high-necked, hook-nosed, white in colour, and dark-eyed; his determination to succeed is tempered by self-control and respect for others, which is to say that he is an ally of true glory; and he needs no whip, but is guided only by spoken commands. The other is crooked, over-large, a haphazard jumble of limbs; he has a thick, short neck, and a flat face; he is black in colour, with grey, bloodshot eyes, an ally of excess and affectation, hairy around the ears, hard of hearing, and scarcely to be controlled with a combination of whip and goad.[16]

The Greeks took it as natural that beautiful boys excite lust in men, and the drama begins when this equipage comes in sight of one. The charioteer, who is usually thought to be the emblem of reason, nevertheless finds that "his whole soul is suffused with a sensation of heat, and he is filled with the tingling and pricking of desire." The black horse, lust, compels them to head toward the boy, and to "bring up the subject of the pleasures of sex." But the charioteer sees only true beauty, which he imagines on a pedestal next to self-control. So he "rears back in awe" and brings down both horses. The good horse "drenched in shame and horror," doesn't seem to mind this apparent setback, but the black horse breaks out into furious abuse and plunges forward, repeating the drama again and again. After enough of this, however, it becomes tamed, and "when it sees the good-looking boy, it is frightened to death, and the upshot is that at last the lover's soul follows his beloved in reverence and awe."

This is hot stuff, but it is only the first act. Eventually the boy's soul in turn starts to fill with love, to "see himself in his lover as in a mirror," and eventually he is inclined "not to refuse any request the lover might make." And then there is a choice. If the better parts of their minds win, they live a life of self-control, since they have "enslaved the part which allowed evil into the soul and freed the part which allowed goodness in." They are then well on the way to immortality. But if they live a more ordinary life ("devoted to prestige rather than to philosophy"), then they will "choose the course which is considered the most wonderful of all by the common run of mankind, and consummate their relationship." This is not too bad, although it will not be "approved of by their whole minds." In particular, it does not damn them for good: love is always the start of a skyward journey, even when the bad horse gets its lustful way. There is no suggestion that either the lover or the boy is particularly polluted by the act. We are far from a world in which they need counseling or prison. Indeed, a peculiarity of the picture is that if the couple want to gain prestige rather than become philosophers, they will go at it rather than restrain themselves.

On the other hand, there is ambivalence and even anxiety in the air. In fact, as Michel Foucault has emphasized, there was a definite script for what was expected in this kind of relationship.[17] The man would feel pleasure, but the boy would not; the boy could submit only after a decent interval of courtship, and not too often; the boy would need a nonsexual motive, and this would be what the man could offer him by way of a road to citizenship: education, or connections and influence. It would be dishonorable, for example, for the boy to acquiesce simply for money.

As far as the theory of mind and motivation goes, there are a number of puzzles in Plato's metaphor. What role does the white horse play, since it seems to do nothing but side with the charioteer? The conflict seems to be a simple two-sided one, between lust and something like honor or shame, so a better image might have been of two horses tugging the opposite ends of a rope. And what motivates the charioteer himself? He is the embodiment of reason, but also the locus of the original emotions, the tingling and prickings of desire, for it is explicit that he himself, and not only the black horse, feels those.

These problems may be the inevitable fate of "homuncular" models of the mind. These are models that think of separate faculties, such as reason, pleasure, or desire, in terms of little agents within us competing or cooperating for control of us. These little agents then turn out to be themselves amalgams of the faculties—reason desires, and desire reasons—and we are no farther on in understanding reason, desire, and self-control.

Perhaps Plato's purpose is not affected by these problems. He is conceptualizing the mind on a parallel with his two favorite examples of social organization: the city and the family. Each of these can be run in justice and harmony, and each can fall catastrophically short. The abuse of power was a permanent anxiety for Greek politics: the unbridled lusts of a tyrant literally destroyed cities and caused revolutions.

For our purposes, what is clear is that poor lust is already firmly categorized: misshapen, deaf to entreaty, and above all shameful. The context is not Christian in the least, but the presumption is not only that lust is willful and therefore in need of restraint, for the same could be said of any appetite, such as the desire for food; the further presumption is that lust is shameful, and that to succumb to the pleasures of sexuality is intrinsically some kind of failure. What was the argument for this? It seems to have crept in simply as an axiom that we are all to rely upon. Yet at the same time the mass of mankind is represented as regarding the sexual consummation of the relationship as not only permissible, but "most wonderful of all."

In his dialogue the *Symposium,* Plato brings up another crux in the notion of sexual desire. One of the speakers, the comic dramatist Aristophanes, explains the nature of love with a charming myth. Originally each of us formed a unity with someone else, either male-male, or female-female, or one of each, androgynous, as the case might be. In this state each individual had four hands, four legs, and two sets of genitals, and was more or less spherical. Unfortunately this gave them sufficient strength and vigor to attack the gods. In response Zeus, the king of the gods, cut us in half like flatfish. But this leaves us with an intense desire to recapture our lost unity. So it is that we roam around, seeking our original partners. Those men who are cut from the combined gender, the androgynous, are attracted to women, "and many adulterers are from this group." The corresponding women are drawn to men (and are in danger of being adulteresses); and then there are men drawn to men, and women drawn to women, depending on their original constitution. Erotic desire is the "desire and pursuit of the whole."

Although it is incidental to our theme, it is notable that Aristophanes draws the moral that it is not shameful for boys to enjoy relations with older men. On the contrary boys from an original male-male unity "are brave bold and masculine, and welcome the same qualities in others." In support of this, Aristophanes cites the evidence that they "are the only ones who, when grown up, end up as politicians."

In response to this delightful myth, Socrates responds with what he has learned of erotic passion from a wise old priestess,

Diotima. She tells him of an ascent of the soul. At first, when someone is young, he (we might add, or she) is drawn toward beautiful bodies. At that time he should love just one body, and in that relationship "produce beautiful discourses." But then

> he should realize that the beauty of any one body is closely related to that of another, and that, if he is to pursue beauty of form, it's very foolish not to regard the beauty of all bodies as one and the same. Once he's seen this, he'll become a lover of all beautiful bodies, and will relax his intense passion for just one body, despising this passion and regarding it as petty. After this, he should regard the beauty of minds as more valuable than that of the body. . . . he will be forced to observe the beauty in practices and laws and to see that every type of beauty is closely related to every other.[18]

And then instead of his original "low and small-minded slavery," he will be turned toward the "great sea of beauty," and gazing on it "he'll give birth, through a boundless love of knowledge, to many beautiful and magnificent discourses and ideas."

It is breathtaking, but it is still not over. In the final movement, there is a kind of religious transformation, in which the aspiring soul catches sight of beauty itself, or the form of beauty, eternal and unchanging, and such that "when other things come to be or cease, it is not increased or decreased in any way nor does it undergo any change." Plato calls this object of erotic attachment divine, and the staircase he describes has been the inspiration of religious minds ever since, having perhaps its finest expression in Dante.

We need to notice a number of things. First, in all three myths, this myth of ascent, that of Aristophanes, and that of the charioteer, Plato steeps us in the idea that we do not really know what we want, that lust needs interpreting and explaining. In each he contrasts the "true" object of passion with the apparent object. In Diotima's story, the true or proper aim of human beings is only what you get at the end of the ascent. In Aristophanes' myth, the amputated halves do not realize that their restlessness is a search for a unity that has been destroyed, while in the *Phaedrus,* the black horse represents not something the charioteer wants, but only part of him.

Secondly, while we might stumble at the association, in Diotima's myth Plato apparently has no problem in seeing the divine rapture at the end of the process as perfectly continuous with the lust that started it out. The object has changed, but the energy and the excitement have not. We are likely to balk at that, thinking that Plato has simply described an idealized process in which lust is destroyed, and substituted or sublimated by something else. We settled on an account of lust as the active and excited desire for the pleasures of sexual activity, and Diotima's staircase is more about putting that behind us than about merely changing the direction of our lust.

In fact, Plato himself is ambivalent. In the dialogue itself, this high-flown story is followed dramatically by the entry of the drunken Alcibiades, a beautiful and somewhat promiscuous young man, a bit of a tart, who tells the company how, when he thought he had carefully seduced Socrates and got him into bed, Socrates displayed the most stony indifference and simply went to sleep. This might be read as a partial recantation on Plato's part, a recognition that sexual pleasure is a pleasure of the senses, and that in sexual activity the senses respond to the person with us here and now, rather than merely to ideas in the mind (which is not to deny that ideas in the mind play their part, as we shall discover). The ideal partner is not someone with his or her head permanently in the clouds. Or, it may be a reminder that it is individuals who make love with other individuals, and that contemplating such abstractions as a bodily beauty that may be in common to a number of individuals is something very different, and from the point of view of someone wriggling beside you in bed, something distinctly inferior.[19] But it is not clear that Plato means this, for after all Socrates simply went to sleep. If he had started adoring Alcibiades' beauty instead, things might have burst into flame. A religious devotion to abstractions interferes with a man's aptitude for everyday sexual collisions, but sensual concentration on beauty does not.

There is no implication in Plato that either desire or pleasure is in itself to be destroyed or uprooted, or is by itself the cause of calamity and disaster. There are ideas related to this, but they are subtly different. First, there is the idea that desire is always in danger of becoming too much. So it needs control—the harmonious soul, like the harmonious city, is that in which we are in control of lust, not enslaved by it. Second, this implies that there is nothing fatally wrong with the desires themselves. The ruler of a city must control the lower orders, but not exterminate them. The charioteer needs his horses. But third, there is a ranking of higher and lower, and there is the danger of shame and dishonor. Lust is fine in its place, but is to be looked on with shame and even horror outside that place. The Greeks liked to paint satyrs, half-human and half-horse or mule, usually in states of erection, and frequently pouncing upon sleeping maenads, on their drinking vessels (fig. 4). But the imagery of their being only half-human suggests that they represent something marginal, boundaries that should not be crossed, transgressions that human beings themselves should not make, however alluring the activities that are depicted.[20]

CHAPTER FOUR

Stiff Upper Lips

Perhaps partly in reaction to Plato's high-mindedness, at least one subsequent Greek school of philosophy was more matter-of-fact about lust. The Cynics ("dog philosophers") thought too much song and dance was made about the whole thing. Diogenes thought that sex was most conveniently dealt with by masturbation, which is easier than relying on other people: as Oscar Wilde later said, "cleaner, more efficient, and you meet a better class of person."[21] But Diogenes took the further shocking step of arguing that no shame attached to the act, and hence no shame attached to doing it in public, which he promptly illustrated by repeated street performances. Rising to the challenge, Diogenes' pupil Crates and his wife Hipparchia are credibly reported to have copulated first on the steps of the temple as they got married, and thereafter repeatedly and happily in public.

Although it is a digression, it is pleasant to record that centuries later Saint Augustine, quite capable of swallowing miracles in other contexts, rejected this account:

> It is true that there is a story that Diogenes once made an exhibition of himself by putting this theory into practice, because he imagined that his school of philosophy would gain more publicity if its indecency were more startlingly impressed on the memory of mankind. However, the Cynics did not continue this practice, and modesty, which makes men feel shame before their fellows, prevailed over error— the mistaken idea that men should make it their ambition to resemble dogs.
>
> Hence I am inclined to think that even Diogenes himself, and the others about whom this story is told, merely went through the motions of lying together before the eyes of men who had no means of knowing what was really going on under the philosopher's cloak.[22]

In a delicious further twist the seventeenth-century skeptic, Pierre Bayle, in turn quoted yet another philosopher, La Mothe le Vayer, criticizing Augustine for this lack of faith:

How could so great a man allow himself the Liberty of diving into those Cynical Secrets? How could St. Augustine's Hand lift up Diogenes's Cloak, to let us see some motions, which shame (tho' that Philosopher Profest to have none) Made him hide with his own Cloak?[23]

Bayle pursues the issue. Diogenes might have argued, he says, that if it is lawful to know one's wife, then it is lawful to know her in public. But this, he replies, is a wretched sophism, for there are things which are good or evil according to time and place and circumstance. However, he allows that this does not settle the question whether we are obliged to be ashamed of doing the deed in public. If it were an offense against nature, then we might expect that animals, "which so faithfully follow the Instincts of Nature," would "seek Shades and dark Recesses for the work of Multiplication," which we know is not the case. And in any case, many people in the Indies propagate in the eyes of all the world. If we reply that this is all very well for barbarous nations, but not for civilized ones, then we have to reflect that barbarous nations have departed less from the paths of nature than others, like ourselves, who have put themselves under "the Arbitrary Yoke of Customs, and the Opinion of [their] Fellow-Citizens."

Bayle finds he cannot think of an argument against Diogenes and Crates, and turns to lamenting the infirmities of human reason, which is "wavering and supple, and which turns every way like a Weather-Cock." For just look how the Cynics make use of it to justify their abominable impudence! But he still doesn't let the matter go, since even if the Cynics were "incivil, ill-bred, and ill Observers of Fashions," this should not make them criminals. Nor can he find that the moral philosophers of the church, the casuists, have ever found reason in scripture for a condemnation of their actions.

After enjoying himself thoroughly by failing to find a decent argument against indecency, Bayle bows out, admitting that some might think the whole thing rather indelicate. But he defends himself with the standard argument of tabloid editors and other purveyors of stuff designed to tickle us with the pleasures of feeling shocked: "I desire the Reader to observe, that when infamous Actions are but faintly represented, they do not so strongly produce the Horror and Indignation they deserve." Quite right.

We look at shame later. But returning to our theme, in the Graeco-Roman world the next calamity to befall lust was the emergence of Stoicism (although Bayle laments at the very end of his discussion that in spite of the Stoics having very sublime ideals of morality, they nevertheless did not disapprove of the "beastly obscenities" of Diogenes).

The Stoic motto in general is "Do not disturb": to live well we must avoid being carried away by unruly eruptions into the life of reason. Emotions that threaten self-control, such as panic, or anger, or grief, or lust, are the enemies, but Stoic self-command enables us to overcome them. Returning to Plato's image, the Stoic charioteer pretty much starves his horses to death, aiming, like a Buddhist, at a life free from care and concern, a life of stark insensibility. At least, he certainly starves the black horse. It is not so clear what happens to the white one: in the *Phaedrus,* it seemed to represent a sense of shame and honor, and certainly by the Roman period the Stoics were well developed in that direction. It is no accident that the Stoics anticipated nineteenth-century British empire builders with their stiff upper lips. Both had to be careful of their public personas. In each case the dignity of office and the decorum of its occupants demanded an inner control and outward signs of it, a visible gravity showing that the possessor is above the reach of mere happenstance.

Above all, proper decorum includes suppressing any disturbance such as might accompany the desire for pleasure. Indeed for the Roman philosopher and statesman Seneca, whose motto was "nothing for pleasure's sake," the overcoming of sexual pleasure was the crucial step:

> if you consider sexual desire to have been given to man, not for
> the gratification of pleasure, but for the continuation of the

human race, when once you have escaped the violence of this secret destruction implanted in your very vitals, every other desire will pass you by unharmed. Reason lays low the vices not one by one, but all together.[24]

That is from a letter to his mother Helvia, but there is no reason to think that he was being coy.

The problematic nature of sex also infected Roman natural history. For some reason Pliny the Elder hit upon the elephant as the symbol of sexual propriety, crediting the pachyderm with every possible virtue: sense of honor, righteousness, conscientiousness, and above all a distinct sense of shame: "Out of shame elephants copulate only in hidden places. . . . Afterwards they bathe in a river. Nor is there any adultery among them, nor cruel battles for the females."[25] Anticipating a little, we might note that medieval writers embellished the legend with further details. A thirteenth-century manuscript describes the elephant as possessing no desire for sexual intercourse, in this serving as a symbol for Adam and Eve before the Fall, "knowing no evil, no natural desire, no sexual relationship." Konrad von Megenberg compared the frivolous morals of those animals that "live for their lust without divine worship" with the sobriety of the elephants, who copulate only to generate offspring, and Albertus Magnus declared that after giving birth, the female refrained from intercourse for three years.[26] Pliny had only given them two years, but three is more impressive, and with divine worship thrown in it becomes quite sublime.

CHAPTER FIVE

The Christian Panic

It is common to blame the real demonization of lust on Saint Augustine. It is always convenient to have a villain we can name, and Augustine's lurid views of lust and sin undoubtedly saturated the subsequent Western tradition. There is also a handy explanation of why Augustine should have been hung up about sex. Augustine was born in North Africa around A.D. 354, the product of a half-pagan world, and only converted to Christianity when he was 29. Shortly afterward he repudiated the woman with whom he had lived since his teens and by whom he had a son. His ambitious Christian mother, Monica, seems to have been chiefly responsible for sending the woman and son back to Africa while Augustine pursued a career in the church in Milan.

It is not very nice to have an ambitious mother, and to dump a partner and son because of the mother's nagging. So, in this story, pangs of conscience then overcame Augustine to such an extent that he had to displace his guilt onto the evil pleasures deriving from the sexual act itself. Walking in a garden in Milan, he found Paul's Epistle to the Romans: "Let us walk honestly, as in the day; not in rioting and drunkenness, not in chambering and wantonness, not in strife and envying . . . make not provision for the flesh to fulfil the lusts thereof"(13:13–14). Impressed by the relevance of this, the story goes, he developed a phobia of his previous chambering and wantonness, and to justify that invented a monstrous theology based on the concept of original sin and its transmission from Adam down through the whole of humanity, all corrupted by the sinfulness of lust. And just as sin trickles down through all of us from Adam's Fall, so in the Western world Augustine's hatred of sexuality trickled down through the Christian church to infect all subsequent thought and feeling on the subject.

It is a simple story, and some of it is true. But as an explanation of anything it is sadly lacking. Augustine might certainly have felt guilty about his treatment of his partner and his son. But when we describe him as displacing this guilt, we use the vocabulary too easily. Displacement indeed has a role in human affairs: if I am angry at you, but for some reason cannot express it, I may vent my feelings by kicking the cat instead. We all know that it is wise to keep out of the way of people who are angry, whatever they started off being angry about. But if you feel guilty about one thing, such as exiling your partner and child, it is not so easy to "vent" the feeling by feeling guilty about something else instead. Is it even possible? And what would be the function of this displacement— why should it help? If I displace my original guilt by feeling guilty about something else, such as having lustful thoughts, or for that matter having forgotten to water the flowers, why does that make me better off? I am still feeling guilty.

Be that as it may, if Augustine was displaying some uncon- scious strategy of "displacing" his guilt, why should sexuality offer itself as something to feel guilty about? And why should his private psychological problems have caught an audience—in other words, why was the culture ready to receive the message? In any case, the story ignores the fact that by his own account Augustine was well onto a sexual guilt trip before he dumped his partner:

> As a youth I had been woefully at fault, particularly in early adolescence. I had prayed to you for chastity and said, "Give me chastity and continence, but not yet."[27]

The legend also neglects the fact that he came at the intersection of at least three much older traditions of mistrust, some more radical than his. The classical, Graeco-Roman grounding we have already met, and Augustine thoroughly imbibed it:

> Are the pleasures of the body to be sought, which Plato describes, in all seriousness, as "snares, and the source of all ills"? ... The promptings of sensuality are the most strong of all, and so the most hostile to philosophy. ... What man in the grip of this, the strongest of emotions, can bend his mind to thought, regain his reason, or, indeed, concentrate on anything ... ?[28]

The second influence on Augustine was the sect of Manichaeism. The Manichee illumination is that the world was the battleground of two implacably opposed forces, light and darkness. Light, which is curiously passive, had been invaded by the raging, lustful forces of darkness. Light was the domain of the soul, darkness that of the body. But the good soul finds itself imprisoned, trapped, and subordinated to the bad body. The religious life consists in trying to help it to get free, by the usual religious blend of contemplation and asceticism. Augustine later spent a lot of energy attacking the Manichees and their curious graft of Christianity onto the Persian religion of Zoroaster, but for nine years he belonged to the sect. And even more surely than in the Stoics, the place of lust in Manichaeism is darkness and the pit. Lust is the center of our embodiment, the bondage of the soul to the forces of darkness.

The third and most potent influence was the immediate Christian atmosphere. Saint Paul had said that it was better to marry than burn, but marriage was clearly a second-best to keeping apart from the whole problem, neither marrying nor burning. Only a very short time later, ascetic Christian cults were preaching chastity. This, the renunciation of sex, was a powerful outward sign of the changed order of things brought about by the coming of Christ, an order in which a new spiritual salvation was offered. Procreation was unnecessary, given the imminent second coming and transformation of the world. By the second century, the Encratites (after the Greek *enkrateia*, continence, in the sense both of self-control and of abstention from something) held that the goal of the Christian life was indeed an internal unity with the spirit of Christ, and this was a unity that blocked the ordinary unity of marriage, "the most clear symptom of Adam's frailty and the most decisive obstacle to the indwelling of the spirit."[29] Baptism in such sects was the signal of sexual renunciation, the triumph over our animal natures, and a clearing of the decks for a yet more delicious unity with the Holy Spirit. In some sects, especially holy men ritually castrated themselves.

So by the time of Augustine, the cult of virginity was in full swing. For well over a century, many had held that the only fitting life for a Christian was monkish seclusion in the desert. And not surprisingly, if you seclude yourself in the desert lust becomes something of a preoccupation. Saint Anthony, the father of desert monasticism, had to wrestle with beasts and demons, and Saint Jerome tells us what it was like:

> There was I, therefore, who from fear of hell had condemned myself to such a prison, with only scorpions and wild beasts as companions. Yet I was often surrounded by dancing girls. My face was pale from fasting, and my mind was hot with desire in a body as cold as ice. Though my flesh, before its tenant, was already as good as dead, the fires of the passions kept boiling within me.
>
> And so, destitute of all help, I used to lie at Jesus' feet. I bathed them with my tears, I wiped them with my hair. When my flesh rebelled, I subdued it by weeks of fasting.[30]

This in the context of telling a young virgin, Eustochium, how to avoid the "drawbacks of marriage, such as pregnancy, the crying of infants, the torture caused by a rival, the cares of household management, and all those fancied blessings which death at last cuts short." According to Jerome, virginity needs the closest guarding, but even so, by itself it is not enough. There are bad virgins. "'Whosoever looketh on a woman,' the Lord says, 'to lust after her hath committed adultery with her already in his heart.' So that virginity may be lost even by a thought. Such are evil virgins,

virgins in the flesh, not in the spirit; foolish virgins . . ." Paradise is only full of virgins who have not the faintest desire not to be virgins.

Here we have a quite new note, well beyond a Greek caution about the space that desire can occupy and the corresponding need for control. We have hatred, corruption, sin. For the Stoics, an "agitation" may well up in us, but in itself it is neither good nor bad, but guilt-free and neutral. Any agitation is capable of being neutralized by further reflection, and it is the efficacy of this antidote that occupies the moralist. For the Stoic adept, the jolt that comes from seeing a desirable partner, just like the jolt that comes from seeing a bear on the path, is not yet a desire or an emotion. By itself it is of no predictive value, for it is there to be controlled and can be controlled. But for Christians, the first jolt or movement or agitation has become the hiss of the serpent, temptation. And even to hear the hiss of the serpent sullies you.

We have gone beyond the ordered city with the governor, reason, harmoniously commanding the lower desires. We have the need to exterminate and annihilate the lower orders altogether. We need not to govern them, but to use insecticide on them. Even if we manage not to succumb to temptation, to live without an expense of spirit, we live in a waste of shame.

It is sometimes said that Christianity represented a backward step from the healthier attitudes of the Judaism from which it emerged. That may be true in some respects; indeed, it was part of Christianity's complaint against Judaism, vigorously voiced by Jerome and others. However, Judaism also gave us the temptress Eve, and it generally associates sexuality with uncleanliness or pollution. And to the Christians, virginity kept you from many things, but above all pollution. Thus a contemporary pope, Siricius, held that Mary could not have given Jesus a brother or sister, even ones younger than him, because

> Jesus would not have chosen to be born of a virgin had he been compelled to regard her as so incontinent that the womb in which the body of the Lord took shape, that hall of the Everlasting King, would be defiled by the presence of male seed.[31]

In this magical thinking, not just past pollution but the prospect of future stain, even after you had left, would be quite enough to put you off, like being suspicious of a public lavatory not because of who might have been there, but because of who might follow you there.

In short, the association of lust with uncleanliness and disgust, as well as with the wiles of the devil, darkness, the animal, the body, and eventually death, damnation, and hell, was firmly in place. Augustine needed only to breathe it in.

Indeed, in this overheated culture, Augustine was something of a moderate. His rigorous philosophical mind zeroed in on the situation before the Fall. In Paradise, things were as God intended, so how did he intend them? The crucial question is: "Was there sex in the garden of Eden?" At various times Augustine came to different conclusions. He really preferred the idea that in Paradise children might have been begotten by purely spiritual love, "uncorrupted by lust" and without the sexual act. Sexual difference would not have been visible. This is not a particularly moderate solution—it was that of the Encratites and of Anthony and Jerome. But Augustine reluctantly came to the conclusion that sexual difference must have entered in, because otherwise Eve would have been no use to Adam, whereas the Bible tells us that she was. Augustine's line of thought is a little embarrassing to us here, since it appears to be roughly that since there was no housework to be done in Paradise, it is difficult to imagine what other use Eve could have been to Adam. It must have been some kind of—gulp—intimacy. In any case, he relents a little, and ascribes to Adam and Eve sexual bodies designed for procreation, although in this interim view, he held that these bodies would not in fact have been used before the Fall. God would, however, have designed their bodies for procreation somewhat reluctantly, perhaps only because he foresaw that Eve would take the apple, and then, rather literally, all hell would break loose.

But the real glory of Augustine's sexual theology comes next, in the doctrine that *if* they had used their bodies before the Fall, everything would in any case have been all right. Adam and Eve would have felt neither lust nor pleasure. In Paradise, people could control their sexual organs as they do their other limbs. "Without the lascivious promptings of lust, with perfect serenity of soul and body, the husband would have seminated into his wife's womb."[32]

Copulation would have been just like shaking hands. Augustine knows this is hard to envisage, but in a delightful passage he helps us to do it:

> We do in fact find among human beings some individuals with natural abilities very different from the rest of mankind and remarkable by their very rarity. Such people can do some things with their body which are for others utterly impossible and well-nigh incredible when they are reported. Some people can even move their ears, either one at a time or both together. Others without moving the head can bring the whole scalp—all the part covered with hair—down towards the forehead and bring it back again at will. Some can swallow an incredible number of articles and then with a slight contraction of the diaphragm, can produce, as if out of a bag, any article they please, in perfect condition. There are others who imitate the cries of birds and

beasts and the voices of any other men, reproducing them so accurately as to be quite indistinguishable from the originals, unless they are seen. A number of people produce at will such musical sounds from their behind (without any stink) that they seem to be singing from that region.[33]

So the solution becomes that before the Fall, *if* there had been sexual activity then it was subject in every way to the rational will, just as in exceptional people musical farting can be deliberately controlled. Plato's black horse would not even have been in harness. But the charioteer could have done without its tug and somewhat half-heartedly gone at it anyhow.

Warming to this theme, Augustine saw the involuntary, rebellious nature of sexual desire as a symbol or emblem of the whole fallen state of mankind. It was a constant reminder of the original rebellion that led to the expulsion from Paradise. In nightly secretions and emissions, inappropriate lusts, and even the rebellious failures of our members to rise as they should when we want them to, we are reliving Adam and Eve's original crime. The rebellions of the body are constant emblems of humanity's rebellion against the Good. This is the real meaning of the Fall, and of the inheritance of original sin.

The psychological companions of these involuntary stirrings from below are lust and pleasure. It is them, rather than sexual activity in itself, that have to be avoided. The only possible excuse for sexual activity is procreation, which should be initiated without either lust or pleasure. The intensity of Augustine's rejection is illustrated in his reaction to the Manichaean doctrine that embodied existence, down here on earth, was an evil, so that bringing children into the world was in fact a crime, and you should time intercourse so as to avoid pregnancy. Augustine spits on them:

> You desire no children, for whose sake alone marriages are contracted. Why, then, are you not among those who forbid marriage, if you seek to deprive marriage of that which constitutes it? For if that be taken away, husbands become vile lovers, wives whores, marriage beds brothels, and fathers in law procurers.[34]

Eventually we get to a ladder. Virginity is best. After that, matrimony without sex is fine, and next best is matrimony plus pleasureless procreative activity. Procreative activity accompanied by pleasure is pretty regrettable; but worst of all, because it would turn your wife into a whore and your home into a brothel, is to act for the sake of pure sexual pleasure.

It does not seem to have occurred to Augustine that sometimes we require loss of control. We tease people in order to make them blush involuntarily, and we like it when they are involuntarily aroused by our presence or our desire. A similar point arises in a different connection. Exploring the embodiment of Christ in human form, the question confronts the systematic theologian of whether Christ was ever sad. Augustine said that indeed he was, "but sad by taking up sadness of his own free will, in the same way as he, of his own free will, took up human flesh." The trouble is that this will not quite amount to the real thing. A sadness that is chosen is not the same as the helpless river of grief that sweeps us away. Sometimes we can control our grief, but sometimes we cannot. Neither can we switch it on or off at will, and we would be suspicious that someone who could was not actually feeling the real thing. Similarly, a partner who can decide at will whether to feel desire is not quite the real thing. We don't want control. We want to feel swept away ourselves, and especially we want each other to be swept away, just as we require blushes to be involuntary, and it is no sign of shame that they are.

Even in his own time, Augustine had his critics. The most acute, Julian of Eclanum, thought that the whole argument was hopeless. He cites sleep, which overcomes us just as completely, but about which we do not normally feel shame or guilt. He also takes exception to Augustine's view of what is voluntary and what is not, recognizing that while sexual desire is not under the command of the will, bubbling up sometimes whether we like it or not, nevertheless we only act on it by the consent of the will. As the Stoics thought, the charioteer can always rein in the black horse.

There is also a lethal objection to Augustine's association of the evils of pleasure with the stigma of involuntariness. There is no intrinsic reason why Adam and Eve should not have been granted sexual *pleasure* in Paradise, even if everything was as much under control as a good handshake. After all, our tongues stay in or stick out when we want them to, and our lips do not purse themselves rebelliously at awkward moments. Thus we control kissing, but we also take pleasure in it. Surely Paradise might have given us sex like that? Perhaps in some recess of his mind Augustine might have thought, correctly, that this could not really be paradisiacal sex, because one of the pleasures of sexual desire is to create an involuntary bodily reaction in the partner, just as one of the pleasures of teasing someone might be to create an involuntary blush. But Augustine spent a good part of his declining years trying to refute Julian, and in the end, politically if not intellectually, he won.

If we think this was a disaster, we have to remember that Julian's sexual theology was not a bed of roses either. He was a follower of the British heretic Pelagius, who denied original sin only to make room for the possibility of striving for perfection by our own unaided efforts. By a life of renunciation and asceticism we can turn the clock back and regain Adam's original unity with God. Like a good British schoolmaster, Pelagius insisted that we are not at the mercy of forces too strong for our will. Such a doctrine is an excuse for moral torpor. His muscular Christianity offers nothing but struggle. By comparison, being told by Augustine that some things are not under our own control can be quite comforting. Augustine at least gives us some of the consolations of being victims, where the fierce and demanding Pelagius would have us feel criminal. In fact, he thought Augustine was a bit soft on hellfire.

CHAPTER SIX

The Legacy

This is not a history of lust, nor even of ideas about lust. But, leaping forward, we should remind ourselves of the pervasive legacy of the Christian attitude to the body and its sexuality. Thomas Aquinas routinely characterizes marital intercourse in terms that include *immunditia* or filth, *macula* or stain, *foetidas* or foulness, *turpitudo* or vileness, and *ignominia* or disgrace.[35] He also speaks in terms of degeneracy, disease (*morbus*), and corruption. Marriage is not so much a good in itself as a remedy for the worse things that come otherwise: such things as fornication, masturbation, and bestiality.

Naturally it is a short step from disgust at the sexual act itself to disgust at women for inciting it, for receiving the foul male seed, for inciting men to take part in the whole teeming, liquid, swampy business. Aquinas struggles with this, noting that Aristotle himself had said that the female is a misbegotten male, but is unable to follow him all the way, since the Christian God could not have created anything imperfect. Anxious not to depart too far, however, he follows Aristotle in holding that women only arise because humid south winds and frequent downpours produce human beings with a greater water content.[36] He also held that women are more sexually incontinent than men.[37] The medieval church found it hard to shake off the Aristotelian view that woman was an imperfect or incomplete man, merely a kind of passive flowerpot for growing active male seed (although around the same time a Frenchman, one Guillaume d'Auvergne, cheekily raised the implications: if woman is an imperfect man, it follows that man is a perfect woman, and therefore a rather more suitable target for male as well as female lust).[38]

But there is an upside, and Aquinas falls short of the excesses of Anthony and Jerome. His aim was the synthesis of Aristotelian philosophy and Christian theology, and the central Aristotelian idea in this branch of moral philosophy is what is natural for man. Virtue consists in acting in accordance with nature, vice in departing from it. This may seem an unpromising bedfellow for the sexual attitudes we have just described. But the synthesis comes from Augustine, again when we remember the Fall. Nature is not what we find by looking around us now. It is the way things

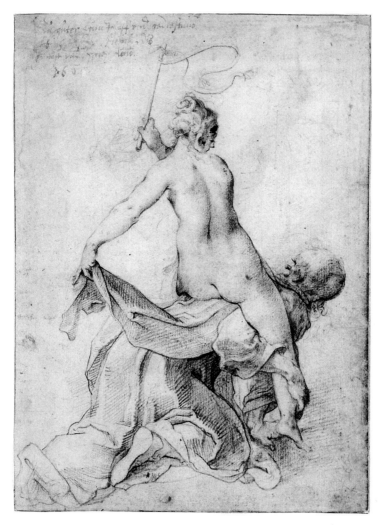

Figure 1. Joseph Heintz the Elder (1564–1609), *Aristotle and Phyllis.*
SzépmüvészetiMúzeum, Budapest. Photo: Andras Razso

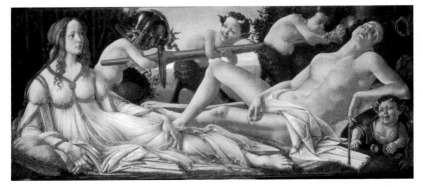

Figure 2. Sandro Botticelli (1444/5–1510), *Venus and Mars.* © National Gallery, London.

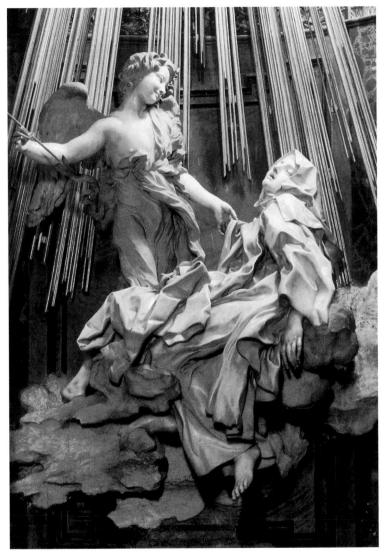

Figure 3. Gianlorenzo Bernini (1598–1680), *Ecstasy of St. Teresa*. Cornaro Chapel, S. Maria della Vittoria, Rome. © Scala/Art Resource, NY.

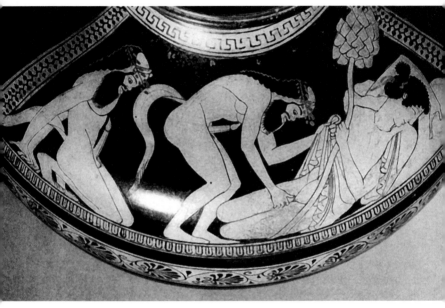

Figure 4. Attic red-figure kalpis representing two satyrs near a sleeping maenad. (ca. 500 B.C.) © Musée des Antiquités, Rouen (François Dugué).

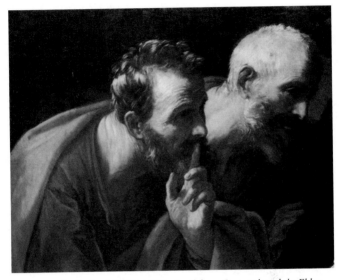

Figure 5. Guido Reni (1575–1642), detail from *Susannah and the Elders*.
© National Gallery, London.

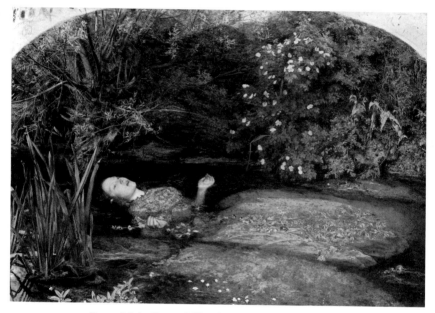

Figure 6. John Everett Millais (1829–1896), *Ophelia*, 1852.
Tate Gallery, London. © Erich Lessing/Art Resource, NY.

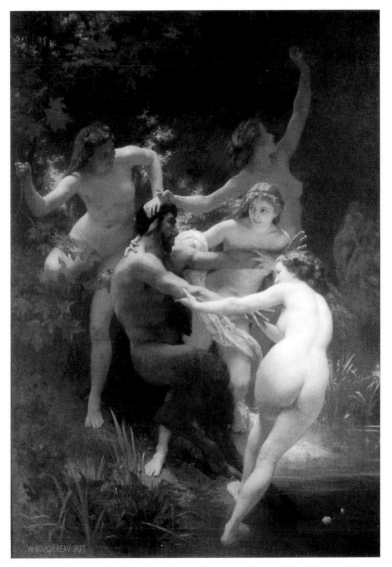

Figure 7. Adolphe-William Bouguereau (1825–1905), *Nymphs and Satyr,* 1873.
Sterling and Francine Clark Art Institute, Williamstown, Massachusetts, 1955.658.

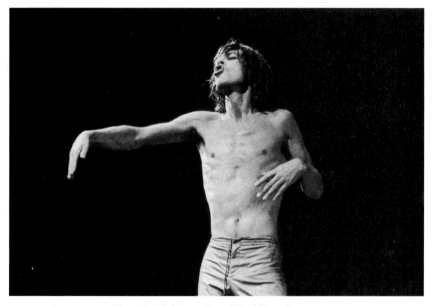

Figure 8. *Mick Jagger.* Steve Wood/Getty Images.

would have been if Adam and Eve had not sinned, unleashing lust into the human world. But what is natural is also what is in accord with reason, and this gives Aquinas a fairly benign attitude to matrimonial activities, provided of course that they are something in the nature of a handshake, and above all done under the guidance of reason. So for Aquinas, "Chastity takes its name from the fact that reason 'chastises' concupiscence, which, like a child, needs curbing, as the philosopher [Aristotle] states."[39]

Is copulation, then, a sin? In his measured way Aquinas says:

> A sin, in human acts, is that which is against the order of reason. Now the order of reason consists in its ordering everything to its end in a fitting manner. Wherefore it is no sin if one, by the dictate of reason, makes use of certain things in a fitting manner and order for the end to which they are adapted, provided this end be something truly good. Now just as the preservation of the bodily nature of one individual is a true good, so, too, is the preservation of the nature of the human species a very great good. And just as the use of food is directed to the preservation of life in the individual, so is the use of venereal acts directed to the preservation of the whole human race.[40]

In a rare lapse from his usual good sense, the great philosopher David Hume said that generally speaking, the errors in theology are dangerous and those in philosophy merely ridiculous. As the modern philosopher Daniel Dennett has put it, you do not have to take out insurance indemnity against getting a philosophical idea wrong. Yet it is almost impossible to exaggerate the effect of this simple combination of thoughts about lust, restraint, reason, and what is natural. The entire Catholic doctrine of birth control depends upon it.

Following through the history, the strictest prohibition on nonprocreative sex soon became central to Christian doctrine. In the emperor Charles V's penal code of 1532, the use of contraceptive devices became a capital offense. Sodomy, incidentally, became a Christian vice only as late as the eleventh century. The biblical vice of Sodom and Gomorrah was probably the lack of hospitality to strangers, rather than any particular sexual practice.

CHAPTER SEVEN

What Nature Intended

We pause to reflect here on the argument that sex is for procreation, and hence that any sexual activity or desire that does not have reproduction as its aim is immoral. Here, philosophy can come to the rescue. The dry way of doing it would be through teasing out various different senses of "natural," and then worrying quite how the move works from what is there, in nature, and what ought to be there, in human activities. The quick way of realizing that something must be wrong is through humor.

The novelist and playwright Michael Frayn, himself trained in philosophy in Cambridge, nicely parodied the argument some years ago when the Roman Catholic Church was debating the encyclical *Humanae Vitae*, which ended up reaffirming the opposition to contraception.[41] He invented a sect he called the Carthaginian Monolithics, who were exercised by the thought that it is clearly the will of God, as revealed by the position of our eyes in the front of our heads, that we should look only in the direction in which we are traveling. That this is God's will is also revealed in scripture by the story of Lot's wife, who was turned into a pillar of salt for looking backward. Hence it is also God's will that when we drive, or what Frayn calls doing the driving act, we should accept its natural consequence, which is *being bumped into from behind*. Interrupting the natural direction of view by turning the head—*visus interruptus*—or still worse with an artificial barrier, such as a driving mirror, is contrary to the will of God, and hence immoral.

All Carthaginian Monolithics were forbidden the use of the mirror, but some liberal theologians permitted the use of the clock, to determine the period of the day (between two and six in the morning) when the chance of *being bumped into from behind* was at its minimum. Others thought that even this was opposing the will of God, impiously averting the natural, intended consequences of the driving act. It also detracted from the delightful spontaneity of the driving act, a thing about which Carthaginian Monolithic theologians and priests were especially concerned. Frayn also noticed that this intense concern was purely altruistic, since none of them actually drive.

Frayn's parody leaves almost nothing to be said, although it alerts us to the fact that in the highly charged area of sexuality, arguments get accepted that would be laughed out of court in other contexts. On that score, it is worth remarking that serious philosophers have attempted to drive a wedge between using the calendar to prevent conception (legitimate), and using a contraceptive (illegitimate). The argument is that if there is someone you do not want to have present at a meeting, it might be permissible to change the time of the meeting without telling them, but not permissible forcibly to slam the door on them. This is not by any means the worst argument in the area, but it does illustrate that when our emotions are engaged, reason goes out of the window. In case the flaw is not obvious, it is that the fault in slamming the door on someone lies in the discourtesy to them, whereas nothing counts as discourtesy to a sperm, since sperm have no feelings to hurt. If there is a nonhuman thing you do not want at a meeting, such as a wasp, then it makes no difference whether you shut the door, change the venue, or time the meeting for a season when there are no wasps.

While we are on this subject, it is well to ponder whether nature apart from fallen humanity respects the view that sex is not to be indulged in except for the purpose of reproduction. In some organisms, such as the bacterium *E. coli*, sex, as a device to get new genetic material on board, takes place, but has no connection at all with reproduction, which is then a matter of cloning. And nature is full of strange sexual behavior, incidentally including a nice version of transvestism (males appearing as females, often in order to sneak in and do some fertilizing when more macho males are too busy fighting each other to notice). Many animals, from marine iguanas to deer to chimpanzees to orangutans, have been observed pleasuring themselves, and homosexual behavior is also common. And many animals, including lions and chimpanzees, have far more sex than seems to be necessary for breeding. A single lion has been observed to have sex 157 times in 55 hours, with two different females. A female chimpanzee has been seen having sex with seven different males, going at it 84 times in eight days (but chimpanzee couplings are quick, and the male penis only two to three inches long). I take these facts from a glorious recent book by biologist Olivia Judson, which should be required reading for anyone who believes that nature follows any one particular script when it comes to sex, including male and female roles.[42] We return to the evolutionary psychology of sex again in chapter 13.

CHAPTER EIGHT

Some Consequences

Before returning to more philosophical themes, it is interesting to chase some of the cultural consequences of the dominant Christian tradition that we have sketched. When something is both intensely desirable, and culturally identified as intensely shameful, we can expect psychic turmoil. Shakespeare gives us Hamlet, unable to cope with his mother's remarriage, seething with uncontrollable images of the filth, sweat, and semen of copulation. In general in Shakespeare it is the villains like Iago, or the deranged and ruined like Lear, who view the world in terms of lust, ignoring the humanity of the world, stripping it down to the meaningless and disgusting jerkings of bare forked animals. Not that we should moralize about lust: Lear equally rails against the envious hypocrisy of moralists who persecute it. But then Lear has rejected the whole human world. The more controlled Iago can see nothing but animal desire in Desdemona and Othello, a desire that will soon be sated and ripe for change. Desdemona will change her affections as soon as she is tired of Othello's body. Love is just a "sect or scion" of lust, merely "a lust of the blood and permission of the will." This is not of course Shakespeare's own view, but a depiction of the disenchantments and fears and jealousies that can arise to torment any of us.

A little earlier than Shakespeare, there was the archetypal depiction of lust in Spenser:

> And next to him rode lustfull Lechery,
>> Upon a bearded Goat, whose rugged haire,
>> And whally eyes (the signe of gelosy,)
>> Was like the person selfe, whom he did beare:
>> Who rough, and blacke, and filthy did appeare,
>> Unseemely man to please faire Ladies eye;
>> Yet he of Ladies oft was loved deare,
>> When fairer faces were bid standen by:
> O who does know the bent of womens fantasy?[43]

Who indeed? Whatever it is, it is clearly pretty bad, since just look what they are drawn toward. Jean-Jacques Rousseau thought the same: "And I really know of . . . nothing more revolting than a terrifying face on fire with the most brutal lust. . . . If we appear like that to women, they must indeed be fascinated not to find us repulsive." This may be why portraits of real honest-to-God slavering lust are quite unusual in Western art. The popular subject of Susannah and the Elders, for example, gives plenty of scope to depict the archetypal dirty old men, but even so they usually come across as more paternal than anything else (fig. 5).

Optimistic, or humane, depictions of lust were possible, even in the Renaissance. The National Gallery in London contains the great Bronzino, *An Allegory with Venus and Cupid* (fig. 12). This picture, painted for Cosimo I de' Medici in around 1560, has had a checkered history. Well before it came to London, restorers had added a veil over Venus's pudendum and a myrtle bush over Cupid's rather prominent buttocks. And when it was purchased in 1860 it was considered sufficiently disturbing that Sir Charles Eastlake, then director of the National Gallery, also caused both Venus's probing tongue and Cupid's nipple-tweaking fingers to be painted over (fig. 13). It was not until 1958 that the painting was restored to its original state, just in time for the swinging sixties.

It is clear that Venus expresses sexual delight and pleasure, along with some surprise, which is perhaps just as well, since it is Cupid, who is her son, doing the kissing and tweaking, and who has plausibly been interpreted as awkwardly bending over to hide his erection (examination of the painting suggests that Bronzino overpainted earlier postures in order to increase its erotic content).

Although the portrayal of lust is itself delicious, it is also true that the bad things that surround lust are here in force. For Venus holds the apple of discord, which lust or love bring equally into the world. In the background is blind Fate, or *Fortuna,* being revealed by Time (Fortune is blind, somewhat as Cupid usually is, because she rewards the bad and torments the good).[44] Joy or Delight strews roses on the amorous couple. Yet just behind Venus is Deceit, with her fair face and her honeycomb of pleasure, but also her serpent's tail. Tearing her hair there is Anger or Jealousy. And in one of the most significant touches, the rose-strewing Joy or Delight is treading, without noticing it, on thorns. Cupid is actually about to take his arrows and go off and fall in love with Psyche, so he is really only practicing or playing with his mother. Like Romeo, his affections light on whatever comes next. His infidelity will enrage Venus, which is why Deceit and Jealousy are so visible, but it all ends happily, as the doves in the lower left hand corner foretell.

Given the times, Sir Charles Eastlake's purchase was certainly bold. Bram Dijkstra talks of the only two possible roles for women in nineteenth-century art: the oscillation between

Madonna and Whore.[45] For most of the century, painting reflects the Victorian denial of female lust. Free from not only lust but almost all human emotion, the women sleep and swoon and lie around in a Tennysonian trance, the kind of enchantment in which all time and all activity is suspended. Sometimes, however, there may be a hint of something draining having just happened, barren kisses, lesbian or solitary sex just finished. Baudelaire is an early voyeur at these scenes, and in England Swinburne followed him.[46] Dijkstra's own classification tells of the Cult of the Household Nun; the Cult of Invalidism; Ophelia and Folly; Dead Ladies and the Fetish of Sleep; the Collapsing Woman: Solitary Vice and Restful Detumescence; the Weightless Woman; and Women of Moonlight and Wax (fig. 6).

But then toward the end of the century there is a reaction, or perhaps a development, not to something any more healthy, but to decadence. Lust becomes the fascinating essence of evil, and woman is its treacherous ally. Classical and biblical literature alike were combed for stories of the Delilah figure, the castrating and death-dealing woman. The headings become threatening: Poison Flowers; Maenads of the Decadence and the Torrid Wail of the Sirens; Connoisseurs of Bestiality and Serpentine Delights; Leda, Circe, and the Cold Caresses of the Sphinx; Gold and the Virgin Whores of Babylon; Judith and Salome: The Priestesses of Man's Severed Head (fig. 15).

In Dijkstra's words, by 1900,

> writers and painters, scientists and critics, the learned and the modish alike, had been indoctrinated to regard all women who no longer conformed to the image of the household nun as vicious, bestial creatures. . . . Woman, in short, had come to be seen as the monstrous goddess of degeneration, a creature of evil who lorded it over all the horrifically horned beasts which populated man's sexual nightmares.[47]

As Dijkstra also points out, in the twentieth century it was not too difficult to transfer these fears onto other degenerates who are supposed to predate on the purity of male Aryan manhood, sapping and impurifying precious bodily fluids, with the consequences we all know. Fear of lust quickly translates into fearful politics.

CHAPTER NINE

Shakespeare versus Dorothy Parker

In Shakespeare's view, erotic love is a kind of overlay or varnish over lust, and what it adds is not itself very much to do with good things like truth and trust. Love is more associated with unreasonable dotings, fiction, madness, bubbles, blindness, and illusion. As Duke Theseus says in *A Midsummer Night's Dream*,

> Lovers and madmen have such seething brains,
> Such shaping fantasies, that apprehend
> More than cool reason ever comprehends.

The lunatic, the lover, and the poet
Are of imagination all compact.[48]

That is, there is nothing to choose between them for extravagance of imaginings. The lunatic "sees more devils than vast hell can hold," and as for the lover and poet,

the truest poetry is the most feigning, and lovers are given to poetry; and what they swear in poetry it may be said, as lovers, they do feign.[49]

The communications of love, the sighs and promises, are a performance. But the performances of love may also be communications and invitations to build.

It is very important that Shakespeare, rightly, goes beyond supposing that the lover is simply disposed to lie to the beloved, as a deliberate strategy of deceit.. He does not agree with Dorothy Parker:

By the time you swear you're his,
    Shivering and sighing,
And he vows his passion is
    Infinite, undying—
Lady, make a note of this:
    One of you is lying.[50]

Shakespeare is more subtle. The Shakespearean lover sees what he or she imagines, what she desires to see. This is why the god of love, Cupid, is painted as blind (it is only evolutionary psychologists, whom we come to later, who depict him as not merely open-eyed but also carrying a calculator). Cupid is also a child, because like children he is impetuous, is incapable of self-restraint, has no conscience, and especially is addicted to play, where there is no distinguishing between make-believe and reality, fact and fiction. Hit by Cupid's arrow, an old self dies and a new one comes into being.

Love's illusions are first and foremost in the imagination. Or is illusion the right word? Philosophy is full of theories and disputes about how much of what we think is due to nature and how much is an artifact of our perspective, our take on things. People have suggested that feelings, values, and colors belong to our imaginations, and only get projected onto the world. Idealism is the philosophy that almost everything is in the same boat: space, the passage of time, our very selves. Various words and images accompany the idea. We can talk of fictions and illusions. But we also have the language of constructions or inventions, which are real enough although equally products of the mind.

If we use the latter set of words, then the poetry is true. We can contrast Shakespeare with Stendhal, who later produced the admired image of "crystallization" whereby the lover projects all manner of imagined perfections onto the beloved:

> At the salt mines of Salzburg, they throw a leafless wintry bough
> into one of the abandoned workings. Two or three months later
> they haul it out covered with a shining deposit of crystals. The
> smallest twig, no bigger than a tom-tit's claw, is studded with a
> galaxy of scintillating diamonds. The original branch is no
> longer recognizable.
>
> What I have called crystallization is a mental process which
> draws from everything that happens new proofs of the perfec-
> tion of the loved one.[51]

This sounds nice for the loved one, although Stendhal's image
seems a little overdone to me. If a partner sings out of tune, the
lover does not so much hear it as in tune, as finds it strangely
untroubling. Lovers are not literally blind. They do see each
others' cellulite, warts, and squints, but the strange thing is that
they do not mind them and may even find them enchanting.
Hume put it like this (the appetite of generation is the sexual
appetite):

> The appetite of generation, when confin'd to a certain degree,
> is evidently of the pleasant kind, and has strong connexion with
> all the agreeable emotions. Joy, mirth, vanity and kindness are
> all incentives to this desire; as well as music, dancing, wine, and
> good cheer. One who is inflamed with lust, feels at least a

momentary kindness towards the object of it, and at the same time fancies her more beautiful than ordinary.[52]

It is nice to be thought better than we are; indeed a lot of human effort goes into appearing better and more beautiful than we are.

Shakespeare stands in contrast with Stendhal and Hume in noticing that it is not only that the lover's vision is clouded. His or her sense of self is affected just as dramatically. The poetry and the performance show the lover not only making up the object of desire, but also making himself or herself up in their own imagination, in something of the same way that people are said to brace themselves when they look at flying buttresses, and to rock to and fro when they imagine being at sea. The poetry or feigning can take over the self, and for the moment at least we are what we imagine ourselves to be. He and she swear eternal truth, and in their imaginations they are, for the moment, eternally faithful. They swear never to look at anyone else, and neither would they, were they always as they now imagine themselves to be. When things go wrong, it may be unduly severe to charge the lover with making lying promises, because at the time of making there was no definite self other than the one in whom the promise was sincere, and no definite intention need have been misrepresented by the promise. A faithful self was being constructed, even if it later fell down.

The performance can bring about its own truth, and evolutionarily this may be the function of romantic love. The imagining is in part a fixing of the self and of a decision, and the communication is in part a request for a like decision from someone else. If all goes well, the play becomes the reality; the poem becomes true.

All this talk of poetry and feignings raises the question of whether we should not prefer to take our lust neat, without the fantasies and crystallizations of love. Conventional wisdom gives us that lust is just about all right, provided the partners love one another. But if it is a choice between lust plus illusions, or straight lust, it is not obvious why anyone should prefer the first. Indeed, the admirably rational classical philosophers Epicurus and Lucretius did not prefer it. What they really mistrusted was love, because love is a kind of madness and overcomes the rational soul. Lucretius warns that being in love entails distress, frenzy, and gloom. If you feel it coming on, you should distract your attention at once by releasing your lust, which means having sex indiscriminately. Lust is better, and indeed an excellent medicine against love. True to this creed, Epicurus was widely supposed to have made frequent use of prostitutes. In Shakespeare the same remedy is urged by Romeo's friend Benvolio at the beginning of the play, after Romeo's extravagant declaration of love for Juliet's precursor:

ROMEO:	O teach me how I should forget to think!
BENVOLIO:	By giving liberty unto thine eyes.
	Examine other beauties.[53]

Benvolio's down-to-earth advice is good only up to a point, because almost immediately Romeo examines Juliet, and we know the rest. Romeo is not cured of love, but simply dumps it somewhere else, crystallizing poor Juliet.

In spite of sonnet 129 with which we began, Shakespeare is by no means consistently a critic of lust. In general, and certainly in the love comedies, love is a class thing. The upper classes deck themselves out with it, but the earthy lower classes (the "country copulatives") have a more robust attitude. Perhaps the best summary is given by Rosalind in *As You Like It:*

> for your brother and my sister no sooner met but they looked; no sooner looked but they loved; no sooner loved but they sighed; no sooner sighed but they asked one another the reason; no sooner knew the reason but they sought the remedy; and in these degrees have they made a pair of stairs to marriage, which they will climb incontinent, or else be incontinent before marriage. They are in the very wrath of love, and they will together. Clubs cannot part them.[54]

Here there is no false sentiment separating love and lust. Of course, Shakespeare is partly sending up the convention of "love at first sight." It cannot be seriously thought that the lovers have really *detected* a whole bundle of virtues and perfections in each other. At best they can have detected a pleasing shape, a reciprocal interest. They have projected or imagined the rest. They have needs that will be met come what may, and under their pressure they fantasize that they have discovered the ideal, the one who in Aristophanes' myth will make them whole again.

One thanks heaven for Rosalind when one reads some more leaden approaches to the same phenomena. For instance, we can read that "social psychological conceptualizations of romantic love have been sexless until relatively recently. . . . love it was assumed was nothing more than a form of intense interpersonal attraction, a sort of liking run wild."[55] We also read that even now, earnest questionnaires find that 65 percent of undergraduates thought sexual desire was a typical characteristic of being in love, which still leaves 35 percent who do not. One wonders what they do think.

CHAPTER TEN

Hobbesian Unity

Which brings us to the heart of the matter, and the issues that separate pessimists about sexual desire from optimists. We said that lust was the active and excited desire for the pleasures of sexual activity, leaving it unsettled what these pleasures are. The best clue comes from the seventeenth-century philosopher Thomas Hobbes, famous for the bleak view of the state of nature as the war of all against all, but who nevertheless wrote:

> The appetite which men call LUST . . . is a sensual pleasure, but not only that; there is in it also a delight of the mind: for it consisteth of two appetites together, to please, and to be pleased; and the delight men take in delighting, is not sensual, but a

pleasure or joy of the mind, consisting in the imagination of the power they have so much to please.[56]

Here things are going well. A pleases B. B is pleased at what A is doing, and A is pleased at B's pleasure. This should please B, and a feedback loop is set up, since that in turn pleases A. The ascent does not go on forever: we cannot separate A being pleased at B being pleased at A being pleased at B being pleased . . . for very long without losing track. But we can get quite a long way. I desire you, and desire your desire for me. I hope that you desire my desire for your desire, and if things are going well, you do. There are no cross-purposes, hidden agendas, mistakes, or deceptions. Lust here is like making music together, a joint symphony of pleasure and response. There is a pure mutuality, or what I shall call a Hobbesian unity.

Pleasures here are not just bodily sensations, although the body will be playing its part. The "delights of the mind" are pleasures *at* doing something. These pleasures involve the idea of oneself, but they are not properly called narcissistic. The subject is not centrally pleased at himself or herself, but at the excitement of the other. Admittedly, it is not just at that, but also at the fact that the other is excited by the self; but this is to be secondary to the perceived state of the other. The mutual awarenesses increase as the body takes over, as it becomes flooded with desire. The involuntary nature of sexual arousal is here part of the pleasure, the signal that the other is beginning the process of involuntary surrender to desire. As Thomas Nagel puts it:

> These reactions are perceived, and the perception of them is perceived, and that perception is in turn perceived; at each step the domination of the person by his body is reinforced, and the sexual partner becomes more possessible by physical contact, penetration, and envelopment.[57]

Hobbes helps to answer the question we posed early on, of why the ecstatic finale can be an experience of communion or being at one with someone else. It is so in the same way that successful music-making is a communion. When the string quartet comes to a triumphant end, the players have been responding and adjusting to each other delicately for the entire performance. No wonder there is a sense of communion on completion. Some philosophers have thought of sex as if it were something like an excited conversation, but that implies more control than should be expected.[58] In conversations we can branch out in all directions, and we devote conscious thought to what we say. Such a model misses out the domination by the body. So in general, a better comparison is to music-making, where the reciprocal sensitivities can be more or less unconscious, and also for that matter where difficulties such as timing are perhaps more salient.

Hobbes also explains why the communion in sex has a better chance of being real than communion with the divine. Conversations with the divine tend to be more one-sided, and some of us think it is an illusion that there is a conversation going on at all.

An extremely important point about Hobbesian unity is that it can be what philosophers call "variably realized." That is, as with a conversation, there is no one way of doing it. This is why sex manuals are so dreadful, except perhaps for unfortunates who do not have a clue anyway, and who need the equivalent of *69 Ways To Have a Conversation* (there are even books that are the equivalent of *69 Ways to Have a Conversation with Yourself,* or so one deduces from subtitles such as *The Secret World at Your Fingertips* or *A Hand in the Bush*). This is also why the "scientific" discipline of sexology, the kind of research that culminated in the Kinsey reports, misses the point, in the same way that an analysis of a conversation conducted with stopwatch and calipers would miss the point. It is not the movements, but the thought behind them, that matter to lust. The way the symphony unfolds can be anatomically as various as the partners can desire or manage, and as psychologically various as well.

Unlike Aristophanes' unity, a metaphysical fusion of two distinct persons, Hobbesian unity is not intrinsically impossible, any more than communication is. In conversation and music it is not just that I do something and you do something that conveniently fits it. It is rather that *we* do something together, shown by our alertness to the other, and the adjustments we make in the light of what the other does. Bodily contact may not even be necessary. In the Nausicaa episode in James Joyce's *Ulysses*, Leopold Bloom and Gertie McDowell, eying each other across the beach, use each other's perceived excitement to work themselves to their climaxes. Unlike President Clinton, whose standards for having sex with someone were so remarkably high, I should have said that Bloom and Gertie had sex together.

However, there is much that can go wrong. As with conversation, there is the boor (and the bore) and the solipsist who loves only the sound of his own voice. There are people paralyzed by shyness, or who fear to speak because they compare themselves, or dread comparison, with others. There are people who are suspicious, and who cannot interpret each other. And the unity may be achieved only because one partner has been "constructed" or molded by the other, obediently taking pleasure in what the other does regardless of his or her suppressed bent, like the wife caused to pretend to enjoy conversations about football and car mechanics until the time comes when she actually does. But whether even that is a suppression of a "real self" underneath, or the comfortable change to new interests, might be a matter of interpretation. Not all education and change is the loss of a Wordsworthian true and innocent self.

We can imagine we share a Hobbesian unity when we do not actually share one. You can think you have caused reciprocated delight when you haven't, as the first page of *Tristram Shandy* reminds us, when at the very moment of his father's crisis, the moment of impregnation,

> *Pray my dear,* quoth my mother, *have you not forgot to wind up the clock?*—— Good G——! cried my father, making an exclamation, but taking care to moderate his voice at the same time, ——*Did ever woman, since the creation of the world, interrupt a man with such a silly question?* [59]

Tristram trembles to think what check this must have been to the "animal spirits" and what a sad foundation it must have laid for the growth of the poor dispirited fetus that became him. But then we all know lust *can* go wrong, and its trials and strains are the stuff of humor as well as tragedy. There is a nice cartoon of two somewhat disappointed-looking people in bed: "What's the matter, couldn't you think of anyone else either?"

CHAPTER ELEVEN

Disasters

We can contrast Hobbesian unity with Immanuel Kant's account of the matter. In a notorious passage, Kant tells us that

> Love, as human affection, is the love that wishes well, is amicably disposed, promotes the happiness of others and rejoices in it. But now it is plain that those who merely have sexual inclination love the person from none of the foregoing motives of true human affection, are quite unconcerned for their happiness, and will even plunge them into the greatest unhappiness, simply to satisfy their own inclination and appetite. Sexual love makes of the loved person an object of appetite; as soon as the other

person is possessed, and the appetite sated, they are thrown away "as one throws away a lemon that is sucked dry."[60]

The comparison of the used partner to leftover food was there earlier in Shakespeare. Antony says to Cleopatra: "I found you as a morsel cold upon dead Caesar's trencher," and Troilus says of Cressida: "The fragments, scraps, the bits, and greasy relics / Of her o'ereaten faith, are given to Diomed."[61] But these are moments of the quite special disenchantment and disgust that assails us on thinking of a third person being involved with our special partner or even ex-partner or hoped-for partner. It is quite another thing to turn those moments of disgust into the universal aftermath of lust. People do not in general see their recent partners in ecstasy as leftover food, nor expect to be seen that way themselves. Even in a post-coital slump one can go on quietly doting.

In Kant's picture, lust objectifies the other person, using him or her as a mere means, a tool of one's own purposes. It is dehumanizing and degrading, and according to Kant it is morally forbidden, since you may never use another person as a mere means to satisfy your own ends. The other person is reduced to a body part, and indeed Kant calls marriage a contract for each to use the other's genitals, so it is lucky that he never tried it. And as Barbara Herman points out in a tight and compelling analysis of Kant's sexual ethics, if sex is thought of like this, it is most obscure why marriage goes any way toward making the use of other human beings permissible, in Kant's own terms.[62]

Kant could fairly be said to paint an obscene picture of lust, one in which all the emphasis is on body parts, and the human being, the person whose parts they are, becomes relatively invisible. The creature that lusts after Beauty is the Beast (fig. 14). Unhappily, many women, and some men, will recognize his account. Indeed, some think it universal, as Kant does, while others think it is inevitable under social and political conditions in which one partner, usually the male, has more power than the other, leading to an inevitable erasure of the personality of the weaker partner, who becomes just the servant who bears genitals to the service of the other.

Perhaps the most notorious account of lust along these lines is Freud's essay "On the Universal Tendency to Debasement in the Sphere of Love," tracing the way in which the idea of the partner as degraded becomes essential to men's sexual enjoyments.[63] Freud works with an opposition between tender, affectionate feelings on the one hand and sensual feelings on the other. The former originate in affection toward the mother, and remain attached to mothers and sisters and respectable women like them. The latter are diverted from these, their desired choices, by the barriers of the incest taboo, and the disgust, shame, and morality that surround and bolster that taboo. So in order for sex to be any good, the male needs women unlike the mother and sister, degraded women, or women who are acceptably degradable. Men may marry women who resemble their mothers and sisters, but they find mistresses among those degraded women to whom they need ascribe no aesthetic misgivings. For Freud, the full sexual satisfaction that these lower women provide comes from the fact that the man can walk away with his soul "intact and gratified" since, having no aesthetic sense, the woman cannot criticize him. Freud was not to know of the kind of conversation that goes on among women in *Sex and the City*, and his sublime conceit never permitted him to imagine it.

In a nutshell, then, sex is either too disgusting to engage in, or when engaged in, not disgusting enough to be gratifying unless one can make use of one's servants and maids. There is also the parallel problem for women, less emphasized by Freud, which results in a taste for hunky morons, such as coal delivery men or well-hung footmen. Like so much of Freud, this might all sound merely funny until we remember, for instance, how much of the lynch mentality in the southern United States was fueled by white male fears of their women's illicit lust for degrading liaisons with black men.

All that is needed for Freud's picture is the idea of sexuality as intrinsically degrading, either to oneself or to whomever one happens to be connected. He may be right that this sad idea was widespread among the Viennese upper middle classes of his time, and that for such minds, lust's only escape was to wallow in the supposed degradation of sex with the lower orders, but he is hardly right that it is, or has to be, universal, any more than the snobbery it trades upon.

Freud at least sees joyous degradation in terms of a kind of human relationship, albeit one reaching tenuously across the almost impenetrable class barrier. In this he is one better than Kant. But rather like medieval confessors cataloging forbidden sexual positions, feminist philosophers have carefully dissected the forms and varieties of objectification. In a classic paper, Martha Nussbaum lists seven features that crisscross and overlap in different ways.[64] First, there is instrumentality—using the other as a mere tool of one's purposes. Then, there is denial of autonomy—treating the other as not having a mind of their own, as lacking in self-determination. Third is inertness—treating the other as passive, as lacking in agency and perhaps also in activity (as with Dijkstra's sleeping household nuns). Fourth is fungibility—treating the other as interchangeable with objects of the same type or other types. Fifth is violability—treating the other as lacking in boundary integrity, or as something it is permissible to violate, break up, smash, or break into. Sixth is ownership—treating the other as something that can be disposed of, bought, or sold. Finally, there is denial of subjectivity—treating the other as something whose experiences and feelings (if any) need not be taken into account. Following Nussbaum, Rae Langton adds the general insensitivity to the real nature of the other, as when the woman's voice is no longer heard, or the rapist takes "no" to mean "yes."[65]

There are indeed many ways of going wrong here, and we are right to be on the lookout for them. Even without digging into the darker regions of desire, it is undoubtedly true that they structure much of many people's sexual experience. Nussbaum illustrates the dangers with examples drawn from fiction, but if we are to believe them, such figures as Henry Miller and Norman Mailer, boastfully advertising the brutality of their phallic battering rams, illustrate most of these vices.[66] The rapist illustrates the fifth in a more dangerous way, while the "commodification" of women, often supposed to be an integral element in pornography, is captured in the sixth. Too many men conceive of their sexuality like their mountaineering, in terms of domination and conquest, while doubtless many people of both sexes are insensitive to the desires and pleasures of their partners. There is plenty of room for tears at bedtime.

If men are socially and economically dominant, it may most often be they who objectify women. In the brutal capitalist world, it may become easy to think that everything has a money value, and can be bought and sold. But selfishness and insensitivity are

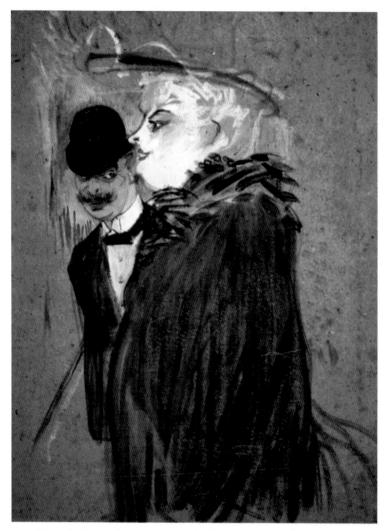

Figure 9. Henri de Toulouse-Lautrec (1864–1901), *In the Promenade, Lust*
(Au promenoir, la convoitise). Private collection.

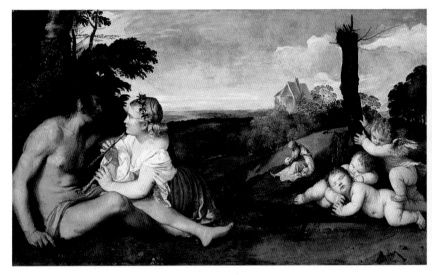
Figure 10. Titian (ca. 1485–1576), *Three Ages of Man.*
Duke of Sutherland Collection on loan to the National Gallery of Scotland, Edinburgh.

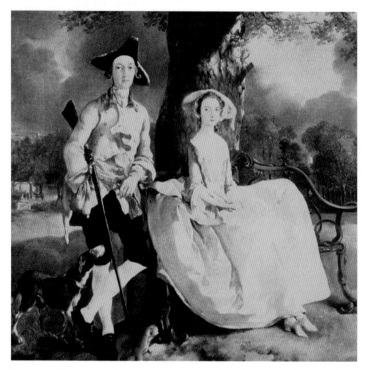

Figure 11. Thomas Gainsborough (1727–1788), detail from *Mr. and Mrs. Andrews.*
© National Gallery, London.

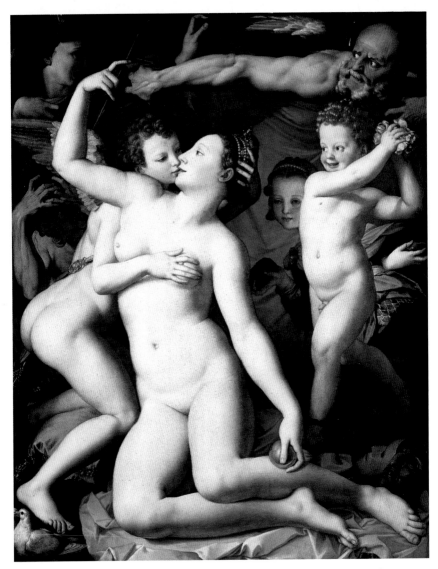

Figure 12. Agnolo Bronzino (1503–1572), *An Allegory with Venus and Cupid.*
© National Gallery, London.

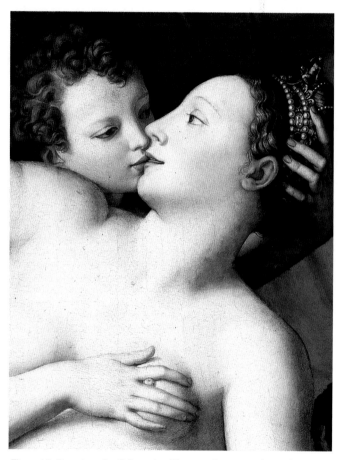

Figure 13. Bronzino, detail from *An Allegory with Venus and Cupid* (Fig. 12).

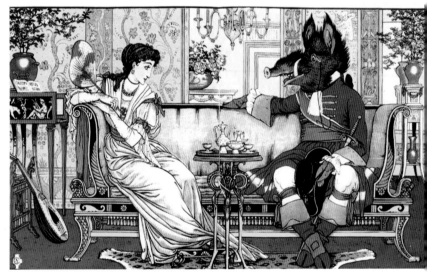

Figure 14. Walter Crane (1845–1915), *Beauty and the Beast,* (Routledge, 1874).
By permission of the Syndics of Cambridge University Library.

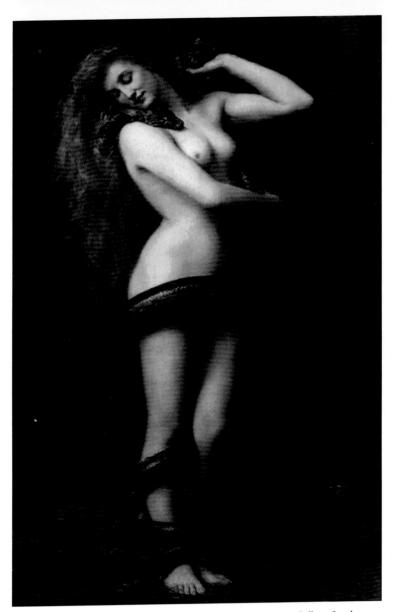

Figure 15. John Collier (1850–1934), *Lilith,* 1887. Atkinson Art Gallery, Southport, Lancashire, U.K./Bridgeman Art Library. © Susanna Greenwood.

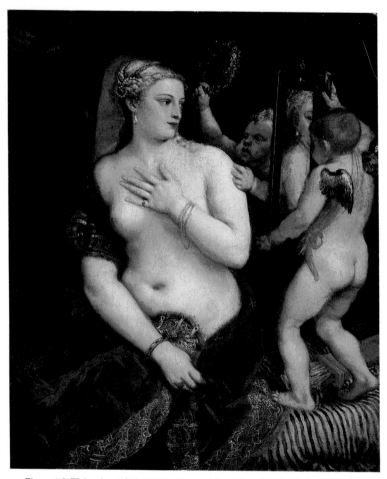

Figure 16. Titian (ca. 1485–1576), *Venus with a Mirror,* National Gallery of Art, Washington, D.C. ca. 1555.

nobody's monopoly, and it can work the other way around. The most elegant, if ironic, literary expression owning up to such a lust is actually by a woman, Edna St. Vincent Millay:

I, being born a woman and distressed
By all the needs and notions of my kind,
Am urged by your propinquity to find
Your person fair, and feel a certain zest
To bear your body's weight upon my breast:
So subtly is the fume of life designed,
To clarify the pulse and cloud the mind,
And leave me once again undone, possessed.
Think not for this, however, the poor treason
Of my stout blood against my staggering brain,
I shall remember you with love, or season
My scorn with pity, —let me make it plain:
I find this frenzy insufficient reason
For conversation when we meet again.[67]

There is a more general male anxiety that women objectify men. The seventeenth-century poets Sir Thomas Nashe and John Wilmot, Earl of Rochester, each wrote despairingly (or perhaps mock-despairingly) of the inadequacy of men faced with competition from the dildo, imagining, that is, that women only want to use men for one thing, and that one thing more reliably provided without a person on the other end of it.

Although the items on Nussbaum's list look bad and are bad, unfortunately some of them are close neighbors of things that are quite good. We have already met three of them: the way in which ecstasy takes over other cognitive functionings, the intertwining of love and illusion, and the limitations of Aristophanes' myth. Consider the first. At the time of crisis, it is probably true that lovers are not treating their partners decorously or with respect or as fully self-directed moral agents. But that is because strictly speaking they are not treating them any way at all, either as persons or as objects. In the frenzy they are lost to the world, way beyond that. But that is no cause for complaint; indeed the absence of this feature is more often a disappointment, to either the person who does not get there, the partner, or both. Even Nussbaum, who is very sensitive to context, falters here, talking of the loss of boundaries, the surrender of identity, as objectification.[68] But it is not objectification, because it is not treating the other either in an inappropriate way or in a particularly wonderful way. The player is sufficiently lost in the music to become oblivious even to the other players. The body has taken over, saturated with excitement and desire. But this is marvelous, even if moments of rapture mean a pause in the conversation.

Crystallization and the creation of illusions about the self and the other also border on objectification, as Rae Langton notices. We want to be loved for ourselves, not treated as blank canvases on which a lover inscribes his or her own dreams and fantasies. We are not even comfortable when put on a pedestal. Pedestals restrict movement, and there is a long way to fall. But as we have already discussed, imagination may be integral to love. Others cannot discover what she sees in him or he sees in her, because they do not share the crystallization. We do not mind a bit of this, and if it is integral to love we can drink in quite a lot. Perhaps we prefer Cupid to have dim sight rather than to be totally blind, but it is also just as well that he is not totally clearsighted.

Imaginings and fantasies can lead people into the kind of playacting when lovers infantilize each other (surely much more common than Freud's allegedly universal degradation). And here again a genuine distortion and flaw may be quite close to something that is a harmless part of the repertoire. Intimate behavior is quite often infantile. Lovers are silly. They tease and giggle and tickle each other, and they use childish endearments. We talk of love play, and sex toys and romps, and play it often is (fig. 7). On Valentine's day, newspapers in Britain are full of personal advertisements along the lines of "Pooh loves Piglet, yum, yum." These may offend against good taste, but they are scarcely a problem for the moralist.

A theatrical performance of being less than a full adult, and therefore happily dependent upon the other, seems to be a perfectly legitimate signal of private trust. It displays that you can put yourself in the other person's hands, let your guard down, and throw your dignity to the winds, and yet feel perfectly safe. The same might be said for more lurid actings-out of scenarios of domination and surrender, in which case the bondage gear of the pop concert doesn't answer to anything more sinister than a desire for safety and trust. Perhaps this is confirmed by the femininity of the dominating male (fig. 8).

Such intimacies are properly private. We would be embarrassed at being discovered during them. The intense desire for sexual privacy is frequently misinterpreted as shame at doing something that therefore must be intrinsically shameful or even disgusting. But the desire for privacy should not be moralized like that. Our intimacies are just as private as our couplings. Embarrassment arises because when we are looked upon or overheard by someone else, there is a complete dissonance between what they witness—infantile prattlings, or, if their gaze is obscene, just the twitchings and spasms of the bare forked animals—and the view from the inside, the meanings that are infusing the whole enterprise.

CHAPTER TWELVE

Substitutions

The fourth mode of objectification, fungibility, is the most difficult item on Nussbaum's list. It is worth noticing, however, that there is no immediate connection between fungibility and objectification. If I feel lonely and would like a conversation with someone, I may talk to A, although if B or C had happened along they would have done just as well. It surely doesn't follow that I am "objectifying" A in any sinister sense.

But we like Aristophanes' myth that for each of us there is just one soulmate, the unique other, and in turn we want to be unique to our own lover. We do not like the thought that if the other loves us for our bank balance, manly jaw, or baby blue eyes, then anyone else with the same bank balance, manly jaw, or baby blue eyes would do just as well. It is a mistake to dwell on the question "Do you love me for myself, or only for my qualities?" since there is no distinguishing the self from its qualities. It is because of our qualities of mind and body that we are who we are. But as a relationship progresses, the beloved starts to gain more and more genuinely unique properties, ones that nobody else has or could have. These are the qualities of having shared experiences and gone through events together with the lover. If those qualities play a role in sustaining the affection and desire, then even an identical twin of the beloved would not be a proper substitute, since those are qualities that the twin does not have. So there is a point in distinguishing loving a self from loving its qualities: the self can change its qualities, for better or worse, but love continues unchanged. Erotic love has the same capacity for permanence through change as maternal love.

Still, it has to be confessed that lust is a little too friendly to substitutability. If we like evolutionary speculations, we might even suppose that it is adapted to be so, precisely to overcome the wholly individual response that love generates. In the play, Gertrude is not given time to have children with Hamlet's uncle, but she is well on the way to doing so. Hamlet supposes it was lust that overcame her wifely loyalty to the dead king, his father. If he was right, then perhaps nature was reasserting itself against the waste of Gertrude's reproductive potential. Gertrude is the victim of the genetic engine inside her. Lust knows no decorum.

One philosopher, Roger Scruton, has gone so far as to say that before sexual desire has the interpersonal focus on a particular person, it does not really exist. So fungibility is actually incompatible with desire. In a remarkable passage he writes:

> Likewise with randiness, the state of the sailor who storms ashore, with the one thought "woman" in his body. His condition might be described as desire for a woman, but for no particular woman. Such a description, however, seriously misrepresents the transition that occurs when the woman is found and he is set on the path of satisfaction. For now he has found the woman whom he wants, whom he seeks to arouse and upon whom his thoughts and energies are focused. It would be better to say that, until that moment, he desired *no* woman. His condition was one of desiring to desire. . . . desire is as distinct from the impulse that compels it as is anger from the excess of adrenalin.[69]

It seems strange to suppose that the sailor storming ashore has no sexual desire. And it is possible to accommodate him without losing Scruton's idea that sex is best thought of in terms of a response to an individual as an individual. The description Scruton rejects is the right one. The sailor is like someone who longs for a steak. His longing compels him to go to a restaurant, and there it is—the steak of his dreams. Thereafter his focus is no doubt entirely on *that* steak, as he works himself into what theologians like to call an I-Thou relationship in which every detail of the steak is gazed at, and caressed with the senses, and admired and savored. But before *that* steak swam into view, he still wanted a steak. He wanted a steak from the beginning: he did not just want to want a steak, as I suppose someone very different might, who is worried about his feeble appetite. This was not the sailor's problem. In the sexual case, what the sailor desired was relief from womanlessness. But that can be a genuine desire or lust, just like desire for relief from steakless-ness (the great philosopher W. V. Quine talked of someone wanting a sailboat, seeking relief from slooplessness). Similarly, a person might be just *angry*, while still waiting for something at which to direct his anger.

What is true, of course, is that the sailor need have no desire for the pleasures of sexual activity with X, where X is a particular known and desired individual. But that does not prevent him from excitedly feeling his body's arousal and desiring the plea-sures of sexual activity with someone, and we should not let our disapproval, if we feel it, dictate that this is not to count as sexual desire. Scruton may have thrown us off the scent by using an example suggesting prostitution, but the smoldering young people eyeing each other up in a singles bar are in the same case, and money does not enter in.

We enter here into two very fraught areas: prostitution and pornography. Nobody is really going to say that they represent lust at its best, since in neither of them is there a chance of Hobbesian unity. In pornographic enjoyments there is no real partner at all, and in prostitution there is no partner who desires your desire, only one who desires your money. On the other hand, are they quite as bad as normally painted?

There are certainly arguments in this area to which you would only listen because emotions run high. Consider pornography. The notable feminist Catherine MacKinnon has said that the use of pornography is "sex between people and things, human beings and pieces of paper, real men and unreal women," and another feminist, Melinda Vadas, describes pornography as any object that has been manufactured to satisfy sexual desire through its sexual consumption or other sexual use as a woman.[70] The argument then goes that it is a short step from using pieces of paper as women to objectifying women as mere things, little more than pieces of paper.

This seems unconvincing. If (heterosexual) pornography designed for male consumption is pieces of paper used as a woman, then when I thrill to the description of the battle as I read some history, I must be using pieces of paper as cannon or sabers. Or, if I weep for the poor Countess as I listen to *Figaro*, I am using the CD as an abandoned wife. And then, by a parallel argument, it should be a short step to using cannons as pieces of paper, or abandoned wives as CDs, in spite of each of these being quite hard things to accomplish.

I should say instead that the central use of pornography, as with other words and pictures, is to excite the imagination. What is imagined is a partner, and she or he may be doing things as willingly or enthusiastically, as actively or passively, or as sensitively or tenderly, as the consumer's inclinations run. People's fantasies may not always be of sex at its best, but there is little reason to deny that they can be. Of course, this does not by itself exonerate the pornographer. There are problems of production, and there are problems in the way women are falsely presented as endlessly available, that constitute real objections. For there are many men in whom the distance between fantasy and reality is less than it should be.

Prostitution is not a simple matter, either. If a person is experienced enough or mature enough to realize that they aspire to Hobbesian unity, then they may not be much motivated to pay for sex. If they are, I should describe what they are paying for as a piece of theater. We have already seen that sexual excitement can lead to imaginings that go beyond rational, clearsighted belief, and these imaginings may infuse this transaction. The good prostitute pretends desire, and the client presumably goes along with the make-believe and for a brief while lives his dream. The prostitute acts a role as a character in his play. So at least W. H. Auden thought:

> At Dirty Dick's and Sloppy Joe's
>> We drank our liquor straight,
> Some went upstairs with Margery,
>> And some, alas, with Kate;
> And two by two like cat and mouse
> The homeless played at keeping house.[71]

Sad and touching, rather than wicked and sinful, although the sinister "cat and mouse" image reminds us that both the prostitute and her client are using someone else merely as a means to their own end. Roger Scruton suggests that the institution of the brothel has a function of disguising the cash nexus from the client, since he does not directly pay the woman, and this may well be true.[72]

Of course, that is not to deny that things in the real world are often a lot worse than this. Prostitutes become victims of male hatred and rage, but we have already said that pure lust can be contaminated by things a lot more impure. The reality principle comes back, and the client realizes that what he really desired— Hobbesian unity—cannot be bought and has not been delivered.

And the resulting deflation, especially when overlaid by the cultural baggage we have talked about, that is, with self-hatred, disgust, guilt, and shame, may prove dangerous for anyone in the vicinity. The law, however, prefers to let defenseless young women bear the brunt of this, as of so many other exploitations, so that it can go on pretending that it does not happen.[73]

Evolution and Desire

Evolutionary psychology is a relative newcomer to the literature on lust. The aim of the evolutionary psychologist is to identify universal constants of human psychology, and then to propose and test the theory that they are evolutionary adaptations. An adaptation is an "inherited and reliably developing characteristic that came into existence through natural selection because it helped to solve a problem of survival or reproduction during the period of its evolution."[74] It exists in the form it does because it has solved a specific problem of survival or reproduction recurrently over evolutionary history. It stands its owner in slightly better stead in life, and as a result those who have it gradually outbreed those who do not. Adaptations should be distinguished from their by-products, which are not directly selected for under evolutionary pressure, and there may be accidents or "noise" in the system: psychological mechanisms that have no connection at all with evolutionary success. According to the standard textbook, an adapted psychological mechanism should have the following list of characteristics. It can be inherited, and

1. It is designed to take in only a narrow slice of information.

2. It tells the organism the particular adaptive problem it is facing. No consciousness or awareness of the problem is necessary, but the information generates a response from the organism.

3. The response is transformed through decision rules into output.

4. The output can be physiological activity, information to other psychological mechanisms, or manifest behavior.

5. The output is directed to solution of a particular evolutionary problem.

So, for example, foods that are good for us, or were good for us throughout generations of evolution, taste nice, and ones that are not do not taste so nice. This is no accident: any creatures in whom the opposite is true fare badly. It is plausible to say that the disgust we feel for bodily waste or excretions is such a mechanism. Our nose or other organs signal that something potentially harmful is about, we shrink away from it, and this solves the problem of keeping us from contamination or risk to health. The sickness and sensitivity to different foods women often feel early in pregnancy probably has a health function. It diminishes the chance of the woman ingesting toxic or mildly toxic substances, at just the time that the fetus is forming organs that might be adversely affected by such substances. It is plausible to say that this is why the mechanism exists.[75] The examples nicely illustrate the second condition above. The *organism* is "told" of the good taste or the toxicity, but the *person* may be quite unaware of it. All she has to do is to like the taste, dislike the smell, or feel sick. She does not have to know why. A similar reaction is the well-known specific aversion to a particular food consequent upon getting an illness such as influenza shortly after eating it. The illness may have nothing to do with the food, but nature does not take the chance. It imprints the aversion, just in case.

Although sickness is essentially a state that makes one averse to certain food or all foods, what the person actually does is then up to her. She may despise herself for feeling weak and defiantly try to eat the food anyhow. But nature may prove too strong, and the defiance may end in a trip to the bathroom. Horace's tag remains in force: *Naturam expellas furca, tamen usque recurret,* "you can expel nature with a pitchfork, but she always returns."

Evolutionary psychology has been more controversial than it needs to be, raising specters of "genetic determinism," or of the mind as a bundle of "modules" that leave us helpless as they function away as they have been adapted to do. Evolutionary psychologists indignantly reject the fear, arguing that the mechanisms they talk of need not be rigid, inflexible routines, such as "instincts" were taken to be, but can be highly context sensitive, and in any case may generate only inputs to further decision-making processes, as in the woman who defiantly tries to ignore her morning sickness.

Nevertheless, there are problems in the air. Consider male aggression, a common target of evolutionary explanation. Whatever else it is, male aggression is highly context sensitive. As evolutionary psychologist Stephen Pinker notes, in a few generations bloodthirsty Europe has given way to a notably peaceful climate.[76] This has to be a cultural achievement, since evolution has had too little time to work, even if, as does not seem very likely, the more boisterous Europeans were either generating fewer children, or providing them with fewer resources to grow to maturity, than any peaceable minority. A familiar cultural comparison is that Canada has around one-quarter the homicide rate of the United States. So any "aggression" mechanism must be flexible or context sensitive, giving different upshots in different environments. It would have to be pictured in terms of a conditional trigger: if the environment is thus and so, get aggressive; otherwise, back off. This is not in itself an objection, for after all animals, too, can have routines that are in the same way conditional. A routine might take the shape: if the competitor is bigger than you, back off; otherwise, get aggressive.

Described like this, increasing sensitivity carries a cost to the evolutionary story. The more various the conditions under which different responses are generated, the less likely it is that evolution has thrown up environmental pressure for each part of the mechanism to develop. There has been insufficient time for human beings to adapt biologically to all the different environments to which we adapt culturally. Let me explain. There is no adaptive mechanism specifically for learning English, since a tendency to learn English is not heritable, and English itself has been around for too short a time for generations of children who learn English to flourish more than those who do not. For the same reason, there has been no time for a more complex heritable disposition: "If surrounded by English speakers, learn English, and if surrounded by French, learn French." But there may have been time for something universal to become an adaptation, and it will be an adaptation that delivers the context sensitivity without having had to prove its mettle in each different context. This would be something like: imitate the language of those around you. That works to get the baby's language up and running, English in England and French in France.[77]

Similarly, a complex psychological response delicately tuned to different contexts will not have been able to prove its mettle in each context. As in the language-learning case, it might better be thought of as the result of a general instruction: imitate the levels of violence around you. That may be nearer the truth, for the imitative nature of babies and children is empirically very well attested. But as it stands it is certainly too simple, for although we do not know of babies that grow up in purely English surroundings yet start to speak French, we do know that other imitative habits are less determinate. Peaceable people can grow surrounded by violence; roses grow on dunghills.

These subtleties matter, because they affect any assessment of the significance of alleged results of evolutionary psychology. If the simple instruction to be aggressive is scripted in the genes, then we will have to resign ourselves to designing social structures around the datum of aggression. But if what is scripted is the instruction to imitate the levels of aggression around you, we can aim for a more optimistic outcome. Bring about socially peaceful conditions, and you may bring about peaceable people. If the sensitivity to context is yet greater, then we will need different solutions again. Different hypotheses are all consistent with an evolutionary approach, but it would take a delicate view of human life to decide which ones are nearer the truth. This means that it is unwise to use evolutionary psychology to pursue an overt or hidden agenda of designing political setups, proclaiming limits on what is humanly possible.

Since mating and reproduction are so important to human beings, they have been natural subjects for evolutionary psychology, sometimes to the outrage of feminists, who see the enterprise as a conservative ploy designed (or adapted) to validate a broadly patriarchal status quo. We all know the standard script. Sexual selection by females is very widespread in nature, as Darwin noted, and humans are no exception. Because women's minimum biological investment in reproduction is much greater than that of men, women need to be choosy about offering their favors. So women are modest and selective and need a whole lot of wooing. Men, on the other hand, may be reproductively successful by fertilizing whomsoever they can. They spread it around, for, as it is said, women need wooing, but men just need a place. Women are at their best reproductively in their late teens, being more likely to conceive on any given occasion, and also having a longer breeding career in front of them, than older women. So men fancy hot young bodies with the right signs of health, such as a neat waist-to-hip ratio, glowing skins, and good teeth. Women, on the other hand, need to be assured of support during pregnancy and child rearing, so they fancy slightly older, successful males who can offer them the necessary resources and to whom they then cling like leeches. An "unconscious genetic calculus" thus rules our tastes and proclivities. It's just tough, especially for women in later life, where the alpha male has so much better chance of lusty pleasures than his matronly wife.

It is a good story, especially for alpha male, high status, adequately wealthy evolutionary psychologists well beyond their teenage years. But it runs into complexity and counterexamples. It would not, for instance predict, Helena's devout doting, doting in idolatry, on the "spotted and inconstant" Demetrius.[78] Helena, like other teenage daughters of whom one hears tell, is out of line on each of three counts. Spots are not good signs of fitness, inconstancy suggests there may be a problem about this boy as a reliable provider of resources, and Demetrius is very young and therefore of relatively low status.

The standard story even meets trouble from human shape. By contrast with chimpanzees, gorillas contentedly stay pretty faithful to one another, and as a result the male equipment is tiny—there is no need to invest a lot of energy making more sperm and a better delivery system if there is no competition. So it is plausible that the relative size of penis or testicles in the male is an index of the need to swamp competition, and hence an index of female promiscuity. Human males have large penises by primate standards, and the relative size of their testicles comes somewhere in between chimpanzees and gorillas. These are indications that males are built for sperm competition, designed to swamp their competitors' teeming residues. But you would not need to swamp these residues unless they were there, which in turn means that women find sexual fidelity more of a problem than the standard script has it. If the woman, having discovered the best male resource she can, clings to him like a leech, the male does not need to invest a lot of energy overtaking other males' deposits. But the biology does not bear this out. However little men like it, without a lot of acculturation women may more closely resemble chimpanzees than household nuns.

There is actually very little about adaptation in the standard story. There is no close empirical thought about social conditions in the Pleistocene or on the savannah. Rather, the worst features of noncooperative, fiercely competitive late capitalism are simply projected back, implying the same different mortality rates for rich and poor as we find in the most brutal economic environments today. In other words, it is supposed that there was no equivalent to socialized medicine, welfare, or community child care in those ancient times. The inference is that we are like this now, men and women both, so we were probably like it then, and the ones who were not like this lost out in the reproductive race.

Philosophers tried to explain human traits by thinking about their function long before evolutionary psychologists, and sometimes the explanations compete. Here is an example. In a marvelous section of the *Treatise of Human Nature*, Hume set himself to explain the modesty and reserve that, he thought, were characteristic of women rather than the more forward men. He wrote:

> Whoever considers the length and feebleness of human infancy, with the concern which both sexes naturally have for their offspring, will easily perceive, that there must be an union of male and female for the education of the young, and that this union must be of considerable duration. But in order to induce the men to impose on themselves this restraint, and undergo cheerfully all the fatigues and expenses to which it subjects them, they must believe that the children are their own. . . . since in the copulation of the sexes, the principle of generation goes from the man to the woman, an error may easily take place on the side of the former, tho' be utterly impossible with regard to the latter. From this trivial and anatomical observation is deriv'd that vast difference betwixt the education and duties of the two sexes.[79]

The trivial and anatomical observation is that women always know which are their own children, but men may not be sure.

Hume did not need to know about the size of primate testicles to take it for granted that women are lustful like men and prone to temptation. And he notices that this sets a cultural problem. A crude solution is to institute punishments, including damage to reputation, for female infidelity. But that only helps to a limited extent:

> All human creatures, especially of the female sex, are apt to overlook remote motives in favour of any present temptation: The temptation is here the strongest imaginable: Its approaches are insensible and seducing: And a woman easily finds, or flatters herself she shall find, certain means of securing her reputation, and preventing all the pernicious consequences of her pleasures.

What needs to be done is for women to build a habit of modest reluctance to permit male advances (Hume supposes that the alternative, of building a habit of modest reluctance in males to make such advances, is simply impracticable). But how is that to be achieved? A philosopher contemplating the problem might think it insoluble:

> For what means, wou'd he say, of persuading mankind, that the transgressions of conjugal duty are more infamous than any other kind of injustice, when 'tis evident they are more excusable, upon account of the greatness of the temptation? And what possibility of giving a backwardness to the approaches of a

pleasure, to which nature has inspir'd so strong a propensity; and a propensity that 'tis absolutely necessary in the end to comply with, for the support of the species?

But all is not lost, since culture can do what an individual could not:

As difficulties, which seem unsurmountable in theory, are easily got over in practice. Those, who have an interest in the fidelity of women, naturally disapprove of their infidelity, and all the approaches to it. Those, who have no interest, are carried along with the stream. Education takes possession of the ductile minds of the fair sex in their infancy.

The difference between Hume's genealogy of modesty and an evolutionary approach is interesting. An evolutionary psychologist might suggest that female modesty and reserve was "selected for," since immodest females would be less able to attract alpha males and to bring up children by commandeering their resources, and therefore would leave fewer descendants than their demure sisters. Or, it might suggest that female modesty is in fact a by-product of female sexual selectivity. The woman is on the lookout for the best mate she can get, so she shuns everyone until she is reasonably confident she has found him. Hume gives the alternative cultural explanation. Which should we prefer?

It might seem a close call, but there is good reason to think that Hume has some part of the picture right. In many and various ways, girls are educated into sexual reserve. Consider that many of the most wounding things young girls call each other imply sexual laxity: slag, bitch, whore, tart. . . . None of this would be necessary if evolution had designed the psychology for us, any more than we need to put cultural pressure on each other to grow hair or see colors. When nature has done it for us, moralists can go home. We also see some relaxing of the insistence on feminine reserve, and indeed of feminine reserve itself, in countries where the social and economic disadvantage of women has been addressed, and where women have control over their own fertility. These developments confirm the message of those giveaway testicle sizes and suggest that Hume is right. It takes culture to enforce those awkward duties of chastity, for females as much as males. Hume also predicts that in a social system in which transmission of property through family lines mattered less, the trivial anatomical difference would assume less importance.

It is obvious enough that many people's sexual proclivities have little to do with any conscious desire to reproduce. We have to distinguish the evolutionary rationale for our desire from its overt nature. Lust does not aim at reproduction, but at a good lay. Lots of sex, perhaps most of it, is explicitly not directed at reproduction. People enthusiastically go in for masturbation, homosexuality, elderly sex, protected sex, and oral sex, just to start the list. They are not thinking in terms of genetic investment and competition, or returns on capital expenditure. We are governed by desire, and by Saint Augustine's standards our pleasures are horrendously wayward. Evolutionary psychology has not helped us understand this. A "module" for taking sexual pleasure with members of the same sex would die out after one generation, and the others are not much better.

Evolutionary explanations are also likely to leave us with a deflated sense of our own freedom, making us into puppets of our selfish genes, in Richard Dawkins's famous metaphor. Schopenhauer wrote before Darwin, but what he calls the will of the species is strikingly similar to the "unconscious calculus" of evolution. Schopenhauer thought that with sex we make ourselves ridiculous. But nature has a purpose in so using us. "What is at stake" he says, "is nothing less than the composition of the next generation":

> The high importance of the matter, is not a question of *individual* weal or woe, as in all other matters, but of the existence and special constitution of the human race in times to come; therefore the will of the individual appears at an enhanced power as the will of the species.[80]

Nature makes fools of us. We are puppets of our hormones and genetic programs. But nature repays us with pleasure. The balance ends up just about good enough—who would want it to tip some other way? All we can say is that nature has done the best she could. She generated lust, and left it up to the way we relate to the world— the luck of the draw applied to the chemical or cultural environments in which we grow—to direct its serpentine paths.

CHAPTER FOURTEEN

Overcoming Pessimism

Venus or Aphrodite has an old association with the sea. She is born from the sea, born in a shell. We drown in each other; Chaucer talks of "lovers who bathe in gladness." But the biological symbol of the female is a mirror, which is also the astrological symbol of the planet Venus. For moralists, the mirror represents the essential narcissism of sin, and a high proportion of the great nudes in Western art confirm their pessimism. Venus's narcissism is also associated with her love of luxury (fig. 16).

We have already talked of various kinds of pessimism: that of supposing that sex is essentially tied to degradation, that of feeling ourselves to be puppets of nature, and that of objectification. The lust of the objectifier asks too little, as it were, in seeking only their own private gratification, or merely the Kantian use of another's organs, rather than a Hobbesian unity, or meeting of pleasures. The narcissist, as well, fails in the desire for Hobbesian unity, as does someone who thinks that you can achieve it by paying for it.

But there is also pessimism that comes from thinking that lust asks for too much. The Roman poet and philosopher Lucretius thought this, holding that the project is that of recovering Aristophanic unity, which is metaphysically impossible. The finest expression of the idea in English is John Dryden's translation of the fourth book of Lucretius's *De Rerum Natura*. The whole passage laments the unsatisfiable nature of sexual desire. Unlike the appetite for food or drink, satisfaction is always denied to lust:

> So love with phantoms cheats our longing eyes,
> Which hourly seeing never satisfies;
> Our hands pull nothing from the parts they strain,
> But wander o'er the lovely limbs in vain:
> Nor when the youthful pair more closely join,
> When hands in hands they lock, and thighs in thighs they twine,
> Just in the raging foam of full desire,
> When both press on, both murmur, both expire,
> They gripe, they squeeze, their humid tongues they dart,

As each would force their way to t'other's heart—

In vain; they only cruise about the coast,

For bodies cannot pierce, nor be in bodies lost.[81]

Men waste their strength in "venereal strife," and besides, they enslave themselves to a woman's will. This may seem a bit negative. But twentieth-century philosophers refurbished the idea in terms of other unfulfillable projects. Perhaps lust seeks to possess the other, to incorporate and destroy the other's freedom, to overcome the other. The most notorious account of this kind is due to Jean-Paul Sartre, although Proust can be seen as an ancestor. Proust's narrator Marcel wants to "know" Albertine in a particularly horrible, invasive way, subjugating her entirely to his will, while somehow leaving her as a real person.[82] The contradictory elements in that impulse were given a theoretical embroidery by Sartre.

In a nutshell, for Sartre, consciousness has a big problem with the gaze of the other, the moment when your own subjectivity is itself being subjected to the scrutiny of a different consciousness. In one of his central examples, you are crouched at a keyhole concentrating upon the scene within, when you become aware that you yourself are being gazed at.[83] This engenders embarrassment and shame. To overcome this shame you have to overcome the gaze of the other. The appearance of the other in the world corresponds to a "congealed sliding of the whole universe," a "decentralization of the world." Human interaction thus begins in conflict.

Sex simply exacerbates the shame and leads to the desire either to abolish the point of view of the other, which is expressed in sadism, or to escape humiliation by presenting yourself as an object from the start and submitting to being nothing but flesh for the other, which leads to masochism. Each project, however, is equally doomed to failure, for each involves a contradictory combination of a desire for freedom and a desire for control. At least the desire remains contradictory so long as the other exists. A desire to take over the other person's subjective point of view is in practice a desire to abolish that point of view, to destroy the other altogether.

The empirical, and somewhat horrified, English remark is that while it no doubt can be like this, it doesn't have to be. Very few human interactions, fortunately, conceal a desire to abolish the other (Sartre is even supposed to have remarked that the trouble with football is the other team). It seems so perverse to generalize from the troubled cases when someone does want to overcome, degrade, or abolish their partner, that the exaggeration may only be explicable by some problem with the philosopher. And indeed there is a biographical explanation that Sartre himself gives. Sartre was no oil painting and in his autobiographical work, *Les Mots*, he describes how as a young child he seemed to get by

CHAPTER FIFTEEN

Farewell

So everything is all right. Hobbesian unity can be achieved, and if it cannot be achieved, it can at least be aimed at, and even if it cannot be aimed at, it can be imagined and dreamed. By understanding it for what it is, we can reclaim lust for humanity, and we can learn that lust best flourishes when it is unencumbered by bad philosophy and ideology, by falsities, by controls, by distortions, by corruptions and perversions and suspicions, which prevent its freedom of flow. It is not easy—and we do not side with Diogenes and Crates, after all. But it is not impossible. And when we remember the long train of human crimes that have ensued on getting it wrong, it is surely worth getting it right.[86]

on looks mainly because his mother grew his hair long and treated him as a girl. Then one day his grandfather took him to a barber who cut off his long hair, and Sartre never forgot going home to his mother:

> There was worse to come: while my pretty curls waved round my ears, she had been able to deny the existence of my ugliness. . . . She had to admit the truth to herself. Even my grandfather seemed quite taken aback: he had gone out with his wonder child and had brought home a toad.[84]

Un crapaud. No wonder, then, that the gaze of the other engenders conflict, becoming a source of shame and humiliation and something best abolished. Of course Sartre may have been constructing his childhood in accordance with his philosophy, rather than vice versa, but in the absence of another explanation, the event may be the best we have of this perverse view.[85]

In Dryden, we glimpse again Aristophanes' description of sexual desire in terms of the hopeless attempt to regain a total unity, a fusion of self and other. Since this is metaphysically impossible, we are stuck with an ideal we can never attain, a "trouble" that we would therefore do well to wish away. But this is an invitation to despair rather than a realistic description of the human condition. The "project" of sexual desire is not that of literally occupying the mind of another, let alone that of abolishing it. It is centrally the project of obtaining a Hobbesian unity, which is not metaphysically impossible, and implies the reverse of these sinister designs upon the other. When things go well, what we ask of other people is something that they enjoy giving.

Notes

1. William Shakespeare, sonnet 129.

2. The reference is to the group Confederate Railroad's song, "Trashy Women," whose refrain goes "I like my women a little on the trashy side." I have delicately taken out the gender.

3. Arthur Schopenhauer, *The World as Will and Idea*, ed. David Berman, trans. Jill Berman (London: Everyman, 1995), suppl. to bk. 4, pp. 263–64.

4. David Hume, *Enquiry Concerning the Principles of Morals*, ed. L. A. Selby-Bigge, 3rd edn. rev. P. H. Nidditch (Oxford: Oxford University Press, 1975), sec. IX, p. 268.

5. For more on Crates, see ch. 4.

6. Human Rights Watch, "Ignorance Only: HIV/AIDS, Human Rights and Federally Funded Abstinence-Only Programs in the United States," vol. 14, no. 5G (September, 2002).

7. Keith Thomas, *Religion and the Decline of Magic* (London: Penguin, 1991), pp. 519, 529.

8. The notion of emotional feelings as portraits of bodily arousals is given a good modern treatment in Antonio Damasio, *Looking for Spinoza: Joy, Sorrow and the Feeling Brain* (London: William Heinemann, 2003), pp. 27–133.

9. Sappho, fragment 31, trans. Josephine Balmer, quoted in Margaret Reynolds, *The Sappho History* (London: Palgrave Macmillan, 2003), pp. 1–2.

10. John Medina, *The Genetic Inferno* (Cambridge: Cambridge University Press, 2000), p. 26.

11. Thomas Aquinas, *Summa Theologiae*, II.ii.153.

12. *The Life of St. Teresa of Avila by Herself,* trans. David Lewis (London: Penguin, 1988), ch. 29.

13. *Summa Theologiae,* II.ii.153.

14. Thomas W. Laqueur, *Solitary Sex: A Cultural History of Masturbation* (New York: Zone, 2003).

15. *The Hippocratic Writings,* ed. G. E. R. Lloyd (London: Penguin, 1978), p. 333.

16. Plato, *Phaedrus,* trans. Robin Waterfield (Oxford: Oxford University Press, 2002), 253d, p. 38.

17. Michel Foucault, *The History of Sexuality,* vol. 2: *The Use of Pleasure,* trans. Robert Hurley (London: Penguin, 1986), pt. 4.

18. Plato, *The Symposium,* trans. Christopher Gill (London: Penguin, 1999), 210a–c, p. 48.

19. Martha Nussbaum, "The Speech of Alcibiades," in *The Philosophy of (Erotic) Love,* ed. Robert C. Solomon and Kathleen M. Higgins (Lawrence, Kan.: University Press of Kansas, 1991), pp. 279–336.

20. I am indebted here to a lecture by Professor Robin Osborne.

21. Compare Woody Allen: "Don't knock masturbation; it's sex with someone you love."

22. Augustine, *Concerning the City of God Against the Pagans,* trans. Henry Bettenson (London: Penguin, 1972), bk. 14, ch. 20, p. 582.

23. Pierre Bayle, *Historical and Critical Dictionary* (Lodon, 1710), entry for Hipparchia.

24. Seneca, "Letter to Helvia on Consolation," *Moral Essays,* trans. J. W. Basore (Cambridge, Mass.: Harvard University Press, 1932), vol. 2, p. 463.

25. Pliny, *Natural History,* 8.5, quoted in Ute Ranke-Heinemann, *Eunuchs for Heaven: The Catholic Church and Sexuality,* trans. John Brownjohn (London: André Deutsch, 1990), p. 5.

26. G. C. Druce, "The Elephant in Mediaeval Legend," *Archaeological Journal* 76 (1919): 1–73; Albertus Magnus, *On Animals,*

trans. K. F. Kitchell, Jr. and I. M. Resnick (Baltimore, Md.: Johns Hopkins University Press, 1999), vol. 1, p. 515 and vol. 2, p. 1476.

27. Augustine, *Confessions*, trans. R. S. Pine-Coffin (London: Penguin, 1961), bk. 8, sec. 7, p. 169.

28. Quoted in Peter Brown, *Augustine of Hippo*, new edn. (London: Faber & Faber, 2000), p. 39.

29. Peter Brown, *The Body and Society* (London: Faber & Faber, 1989), p. 92.

30. *Letters of St. Jerome*, trans. C. C. Mierow (London: Longmans, Green & Co., 1963), letter 22, "To Eustochium," sec. 7, p. 140.

31. Quoted in Ranke-Heinemann, *Eunuchs for Heaven*, p. viii.

32. Augustine, *On Genesis: Two Books on Genesis Against the Manichees*, trans R. J. Teske (Washington, D.C.: Catholic University of America Press, 1991).

33. *City of God*, bk. 114, ch. 24, p. 588.

34. *Contra Faustum*, bk. 15, ch. 7.

35. Joseph Fuchs, *Die Sexualethik des heiligen Thomas von Aquin*, 50–52, quoted in Ranke-Heinemann, *Eunuchs for Heaven*, 170–71.

36. Aquinas, *Summa Theologiae*, I.92.a.1.

37. *Summa Theologiae*, II/II.56.a.1.

38. Ranke-Heinemann, *Eunuchs for Heaven*, p. 163.

39. Aquinas refers to *Nicomachaean Ethics*, III.12.

40. *Summa Theologiae*, II/II.153.

41. Frayn's squib is reprinted in *The Original Michael Frayn*, ed. Michael Fenton (London: Mandarin, 2000).

42. Olivia Judson, *Dr. Tatiana's Sex Advice to All Creation* (London: Chatto & Windus, 2002).

43. Edmund Spenser, *The Faerie Queene*, in *Spenser: Selected Writings*, ed. Elizabeth Porges Watson (London: Routledge, 1992), I.iv.24, pp. 116–17.

44. I am following the interpretation recently advanced by Ross Kilpatrick, of Queen's University at Kingston, Ontario, in "Bronzino and Apuleius," forthcoming in *Artibus et Historiae*.

45. Bram Dijkstra, *Idols of Perversity* (New York: Oxford University Press, 1986).

46. Charles Baudelaire, *Les Fleurs du mal* (1857); Algernon Charles Swinburne, "Anactoria," *Poems and Ballads* (1866).

47. *Idols of Perversity*, pp. 324–25.

48. William Shakespeare, *A Midsummer Night's Dream*, act 5, scene 1, lines 3–8.

49. William Shakespeare, *As You Like It*, act 3, scene 3, lines 16–18.

50. Dorothy Parker, "Unfortunate Coincidence," *Not So Deep as a Well* (New York: Viking, 1936), p. 40.

51. Stendhal, *Love*, trans. Gilbert and Suzanne Sale (London: Penguin, 1975), p. 45.

52. David Hume, *A Treatise of Human Nature*, ed. L. A. Selby-Bigge (Oxford: Oxford University Press, 1888), bk. II, pt. ii, sec. 11, p. 394.

53. William Shakesepare, *Romeo and Juliet*, act 1, scene 1, lines 223–25.

54. *As You Like It*, act 5, scene 2, lines 31–39.

55. Pamela C. Regan and Ellen Berscheid, *Lust* (California: Sage, 1999), p. 116.

56. Thomas Hobbes, *The Elements of Law Natural and Politic*, ed. J. C. A. Gaskin (Oxford: Oxford University Press, 1994), pt. I: *Human Nature*, ch. IX, sec. 15, p. 55.

57. Thomas Nagel, "Sexual Perversion," originally in *Journal of Philosophy* 66 (1969), repr. in *Mortal Questions* (Cambridge: Cambridge University Press, 1979), p. 48.

58. Robert Solomon's writings are illuminating here. See, for instance, "Sexual Paradigms," *Journal of Philosophy* 71 (1974): 336–45.

59. Lawrence Sterne, *The Life and Opinions of Tristram Shandy* (Oxford: Oxford University Press, 1983), p. 5.

60. Immanuel Kant, *Lectures on Ethics*, ed. P. Heath and J. B. Schneewind (Cambridge: Cambridge University Press, 1997), p. 156

61. William Shakespeare, *Antony and Cleopatra*, act 3, scene 13, lines 117–18; *Troilus and Cressida*, act 5, scene 2, line 155.

62. Barbara Herman, "Could It Be Worth Thinking About Kant on Sex and Marriage?" in *A Mind of One's Own*, ed. Louise M. Antony and Charlotte Witt (Boulder, Colo.: Westview, 1993), pp. 49–67.

63. Collected in *On Sexuality*, Penguin Freud Library, no. 7 (London: Penguin, 1991), pp. 243–60.

64. Martha Nussbaum, "Objectification," *Philosophy and Public Affairs* 24 (1995): 249–91.

65. Rae Langton, "Love and Solipsism," in *Love Analyzed*, ed. Roger Lamb (Boulder, Colo.: Westview, 1997), pp. 123–52.

66. A devastating, and painfully funny, demolition of Henry Miller is that by Brigid Brophy, *London Magazine*, 1963, repr. in *Modern British Comic Writing*, ed. Patricia Craig (London: Penguin, 1992).

67. Edna St. Vincent Millay, sonnet lxi, *Collected Poems* (New York: Harper & Row, 1965), p. 601.

68. Nussbaum, "Objectification," p. 273.

69. Roger Scruton, *Sexual Desire* (London: Weidenfeld & Nicolson, 1986), p. 90. Although I think Scruton goes wrong in places such as this, I should record a general indebtedness to his treatment.

70. Catherine MacKinnon, *Only Words* (Cambridge, Mass.: Harvard University Press, 1993), p. 109; Melinda Vadas, quoted in Rae Langton, "Sexual Solipsism," *Philosophical Topics* 23 (1995): 149–87.

71. W. H. Auden, "Master and Boatswain," *Selected Poems*, ed. Edward Mendelson (New York: Vintage, 1979), p. 144.

72. Scruton, *Sexual Desire*, p. 156

73. The Roman Catholic church distinguishes itself on this issue as well. Opus Dei member Dr. Clementina Meregalli Anzilotti: "Sexual harrassment comes to those who want it. Some women go around dressed in such a way that they attract that kind of approach."

74. David M. Buss, *Evolutionary Psychology* (Needham Heights, Mass.: Allyn & Baker, 1999), p. 37.

75. M. Profet, "Pregnancy Sickness as Adaptation," in J. Barkow, L. Cosmides, and J. Tooby, eds., *The Adapted Mind* (New York: Oxford University Press, 1992), pp. 327–65.

76. Stephen Pinker, *The Blank Slate* (London: Penguin, 2002), p. 333.

77. I am not here commenting on the contentious issue of whether the imitation needs to be carried out in the presence of innate grammars in order to deliver full-fledged creative and elastic uses of language.

78. *A Midsummer Night's Dream*, act 1, scene 1, line 110. Some editors pedantically suppose Demetrius to have been morally rather than dermatologically spotted, but Shakespeare may have intended both, and in any case the point stands.

79. This and the following quotations come from Hume, *A Treatise of Human Nature*, bk. III, pt. ii, sec. 12, pp. 570–3.

80. Arthur Schopenhauer, *The World as Will and Representation*, trans. E. F. J. Payne (New York: Dover, 1958), vol. 2, p. 534.

81. John Dryden, "Lucretius: The Fourth Book Concerning the Nature of Love," *The Poems of John Dryden*, vol. 2, *1682–1685*, ed. Paul Hammond (London: Longman, 1995), lines 67–78, pp. 335–36.

82. Marcel Proust, *Remembrance of Things Past.* I am indebted here to Rae Langton's analysis in "Sexual Solipsism."

83. Jean-Paul Sartre, *Being and Nothingness*, trans. Hazel E. Barnes (London: Routledge, 1958), pt. 3, ch. 1, pp. 259 ff.

84. Jean-Paul Sartre, *Words*, trans. Irene Clephane (London: Hamish Hamilton, 1964), p. 72.

85. In fairness, I should add that commentators have struggled to make Sartre appear more sympathetic, if more complex, than this. See, for instance, Nathan Oaklander, "Sartre on Sex," in *The Philosophy of Sex*, ed. Alan Soble (Totowa, N.J.: Rowman and Littlefield,

1980), pp. 190–206. For an outraged response to a similar analysis in Roger Scruton, see Langton, "Sexual Solipsism," pp. 168–70

86. Not to menion the long list of human stupidities. According to the *Economist* (May, 2003), the worldwide beauty industry annually sells skincare products worth $24 billion; makeup, $18 billion; $38 billion of haircare products; and $15 billion of perfumes. The market for "hope in a jar" is growing at up to 7 percent a year, more than twice the rate of the developed world's GDP.

Index

philosophers: feminist, 97–100; and lust, 9–11

philosophy: errors in, 68

Phyllis *(Lai d'Aristote),* 9–11

physiological properties of arousal, 18–19

Pinker, Stephen, 114

Plato, 29, 41, 52; and *Phaedrus,* 30–31, 37, 45; and *Symposium,* 34–39

play, love as, 101–2

pleasure, 16–17, 22; and Christianity, 59–60, 62; overcoming, 45–46; of the senses, 38–39; *vs.* pleasing, 87–88

Pliny the Elder, 46–47

pollution through sex, 56

pornography, 98, 107–8

prestige, 32–33

priapism, 16

priests, 6

procreation, 60

promiscuity, 118–19. *See also* infidelity

propriety, subversion of, 2–3

prostitutes/prostitution, 5, 23, 107, 108–10

Proust, Marcel, 129

Psyche, 76

psychology. *See* evolutionary psychology

public acts of sexuality, 41–44

Pythagoras, 29

rape, 98

rational will, 59

reason, 44, 46, 67

religious life, 52

religious transformation, 36–37

renunciation, sexual, 53, 62–63

reproduction, 71–72, 104–5, 117–19

Republican conventions, 23

Roman period, 45–47

Romeo and Juliet (Shakespeare), 76, 84–85

Rosalind *(As You Like It),* 85, 86

Rousseau, Jean-Jaques, 74–75

Russell, Bertrand, 9, 15

sadism, 130

Sappho, 17–18, 19

Sartre, Jean-Paul, 129–31, 141n85

satiation, 27

satyrs, 39

Schopenhauer, Arthur, 2–3, 124

scientific approaches to sex, 90

Scruton, Roger, 105–6, 109, 139n69

self: illusions about the, 101; qualities of, 104; sense of, 83